# REVIEWS

Browse the shelves of the health section of a bookstore and you'll see numerous titles by well-known cancer survivors and celebrities with cancer, who in sharing their story serve as inspiration to others. While helpful to many, these narratives often set a high bar of expectation that ordinary people living with cancer do not feel capable of achieving. Not so with Eric Galvez's "Reversal: When a Therapist Becomes a Patient." In sharing his journey with cancer, Eric is the "everyman," funny and profound, resolute and unwavering in his desire to live. He has written this book in hope that it will help and inspire others. It resounds with determination and courage, as well as an appreciation for friends, family and life.

-Brad Zebrack PhD, 25-year survivor of Hodgkin's disease


The author utilizes a unique and modern format to present his story in this book or "blook" format. The personal reflections are refreshing, honest and even at times humorous. The flow of the book is excellent and is especially nice for the even non-avid readers; however, don't mistake that for lack of substance, as there are plenty of deeper reflections in the book that will satisfy the intellect. This book is an excellent resource for any patient with a brain tumor. It also has indispensable benefits for the future healthcare professional who wants tangibility to assist with their expectations of their future patients. Not only are the author's thoughts of benefit, but even more so, the family and friends of the author contribute their reflections to ensure that the future healthcare reader can be sure to understand the dynamics of family and friend involvement in their patient care. I HIGHLY recommend this book and its potential in any rehabilitation education program.

-Kurt Biebuyck PT

Reversal is a very unique book in not only the style that it is written in (a lot of quotes from a blog) but also brings in the perspective of a therapist becoming a patient (hence the title). The book is a quick read because it is engaging and in a common language that allows us to really get to know Eric and what he is going through as we share his pains and goals. Further, Eric has been able to do what many of us have been trying to do. What Reversal really shows us is that there is a group of individuals, adolescents and young adults, who are affected by cancer and yet still they lack the comprehensive care that is out there. The clinical trials, biology, advocacy, and even public health issues are often times over looked allowing this unique group of individuals to fall through the gaps of health care and really become an undeserved community. Reversal really allows us to see how this group of adolescents and young adults feel when they and their loved ones are affected by cancer.

-Ali Ansary, Co-founder SeventyK

Reversal is a frank, honest autobiography written in real-time about a young, athletic physical therapist's process in dealing with the diagnosis, surgery and rehabilitation for a brain tumor. He gives clear insights for those undergoing the same life-changing events as he did and also for those treating those individuals. I was struck by Eric's descriptions of challenges of day-to-day life and stunned by different stranger's reactions to him. I know it only gives me the smallest taste of what he has dealt with since his diagnosis, but as a physical therapist myself, I feel the book gave me valuable insight into the lives of my own patients. I highly recommend Reversal for all students entering healthcare related fields, especially physical and occupational therapy.

-Annalee Appledorn PT DPT OCS

"Reversal" is a clever title about a wrestling champ who becomes a physical therapist and then a PT patient, after suffering a brain tumor. The writing is a little uneven in pace and a tad repetitive. But the heart of a competitor and survivor beats on every page. Eric Galvez's story is inspirational and moving. The lesson is simple: never give up.

-Ron Donoho, Editor in Chief, SanDiego.com

I have to say that this book is a necessity for all Physical Therapists (and Occupational Therapists for that matter), and I sincerely hope it makes it into the mandatory reading list for those in training. The author's sense of humor and outlook in life is amazingly positive, and that reflects well in the book especially as he overcomes all of these incredible obstacles. He takes us on an adventure, from the surgery and through all of the rehab that came afterward in order to regain simple movements that we tend to take for granted. After reading this book, I promise never to take those things for granted again.

-Nanette Hale, Doctor of Oriental Medicine

By giving honest and truthful descriptions of various events along his experience, the author does a great job of sharing a unique perspective of a young, athletic physical therapist who must undergo treatment as a patient and then endure the emotional and physical struggles of recovery through his own therapy and everyday life. The style allows the reader to associate with the author personally throughout the book thanks to humor and emotional insight. The additional first-person perspectives of family, friends and healthcare professionals that are included in the book contribute to a well-balanced and informative account of the author's experience outside of his own view.

-Burke Porter, Sapporo, Japan

As a PTA student, I found reading Reversal: When a Therapist Becomes a Patient to be very interesting and eye opening. I appreciated the opportunity to experience a physical therapy journey from a patient's perspective, and I found Eric's vivid personal account to be very touching. Following Eric through the pages as he set goals for himself – and then struggled to accept that they were too much, too soon – was heart wrenching. Eric's passion for his work and his desire to return to it was inspiring. The way his co-workers worked tirelessly with him after hours on the surfboard was very moving. As you can tell, Eric's story evoked many different emotions in me. Most of all, it made me feel anxious to begin helping patients on a daily basis, and it made me feel even more empathy for those struggling through hard times.

-Julie Sandner Weisz SPTA

Reversal brought a smile to my face and a comfortable feeling into my heart that I hadn't felt for months. This book had me laughing and tearing up on all kinds of levels right from the start for various reasons. Reading about someone so similar to myself who had experienced everything that I had made me feel right at home. I was cracking up with parts like the magic burrito or when Eric was almost to his room but then his towel dramatically slipped. I kept bursting out in laughter while reading nonstop for three hours, and my family took notice; when they read what Eric had to say it brought a smile to their face that was even bigger than mine. Nobody was laughing however when I started to tear up about many of the things I had in common with Eric. Mysterious and random symptoms that came out of the blue, a shocking diagnosis, and emotional friends and family were the three biggest hurdles for me making my connection to the book much more than just a brain tumor. Eric and I are both athletes at heart, and recovery time from medication or hospital visits meant less physical activity. Recovery time and side effects from medication were always horrible for me, so I was glad to read about how someone else related to me about the exact same things. Thanks Eric for writing this book, creating websites, promoting events, and making yourself personally available for young brain tumor survivors.

-Catherine B., "mAss Kicking" High School Student

# Reversal

# Reversal

## WHEN A THERAPIST BECOMES A PATIENT

### FOURTH EDITION

ERIC ANTHONY GALVEZ DPT CSCS

iUniverse, Inc.
New York   Bloomington

# Reversal
## When A Therapist Becomes A Patient
### Fourth Edition

iUniverse books may be ordered through booksellers or by contacting:

iUniverse
1663 Liberty Drive
Bloomington, IN 47403
www.iuniverse.com
1-800-Authors (1-800-288-4677)

Because of the dynamic nature of the Internet, any Web addresses or links contained in this book may have changed since publication and may no longer be valid. The views expressed in this work are solely those of the author and do not necessarily reflect the views of the publisher, and the publisher hereby disclaims any responsibility for them.

ISBN: 978-1-4502-2428-4 (sc)
ISBN: 978-1-4502-2429-1 (ebk)

For more information about the author please visit www.ericgalvezdpt.com.

Printed in the United States of America
iUniverse rev. date: 05/27/2010

This book is dedicated to my family and friends that stood by me during this difficult time especially my mom and dad who had to put up with my stubborn attitude. The book is also dedicated to healthcare students and all patients that are hungry to get back to what they normally do. The book is also dedicated to the memory of Auntie Gemma, Auntie Odette, Lolo Nicolas, and Daylene Auer who all fought valiantly against cancer and brain tumors.

Special thanks to "Ma" and "Pa" Galvez, Oliver, Paulette, Mason, Lilly, Chris Lum, Alvin, Thompson, Dan, Stacey, Rosalia, and Tony for contributing to my crazy project. Thanks to all my friends for reading my manuscript and making sure I didn't sound too dumb especially Trish Curatti, Puifan Gong, Su Valania, and Jenny Tai-Borlaza. Special thanks to Renee Ross for helping to edit this edition. Thanks to the iUniverse staff for helping me get this book initially published because I had no idea what I was doing. And thanks to all the patients and staff at Grossmont hospital for brightening my day. To the hundreds of Galvezs, Sagalas, and Brions out there... I'll make you proud. To my Michigan cousins/family: the Supenas/Thrones, Borlazas, and Sumcads... Thanks for the prayers and support. Please save some lumpia for me. Special thanks to Paolo Aquino, Reno Ursal, Steve Peng, Steve Yang, Anita Tassiviri, Jess Stratton-Goff, Lyman Ng, Susie Gharehmani, Hotel Pan, Mary Maine, Teresa Burdick, Jeanine Bryan, and Janine Ostrow for making sure I wasn't a hermit. Big props to: Jeanae, Gabby, Korry, Lettie, Linda, Nancy, Marie, Katie, Paul, Dan, Judy, Cliff, Kathy, and Carrie for welcoming me back to "work" and not making it feel awkward. To my young adult survivor posse: Matt Z, the Bouff, Ali, Syd, Michelle, Duane, Christine, Maimah, Tamika, Jonny, Brad, Joe, John, Erick, Giselle, Emily, Meghan, Stu, Jaime, Jesse, Stephen, Phillip, Liz, Selma, Kris, and Heidi... TUMORS SUCK! To my Lambda bros at Northwestern, Boston University, NYU, Berkeley, and the University of Michigan... keep making us proud! BIG BROTHER IS ALWAYS WATCHING! Thanks to all my PT school friends: Chris Thompson, Amy Barden, Shawn Krause, Holly Borgman, Anang Chokshi, Tejal Chokshi, Annalee Appledorn, Dan Appledorn, Michael Tiong, Neda Tiong, Melissa Layher, Branden McDowell, Ryan and Heather Luna, Dana Struble, Kelly Miller, Jodi Taylor, Jen Fritts, Jen Orr, Krista Pollard... I still have a Powerpoint presentation I never showed you... hee hee. To my PT school professors: Dr. Darnell, Donna, Becky, Edgar, Cindy K, Cindy F, Jackie, Allan, and Laura... your guidance has been invaluable in my professional development. Thanks for helping me mature. To my high school friends esp: Wlodyga, JJ, Vigo, Mich, Julie, Kelley, Lapham, and ALL my teachers and coaches: Ms K-M, Couch Caudill, Coach Settles, Coach Kneebone, Richard, Mr. Heslip, Mrs. Pezda… see I do talk! The list could go on and on; I wish I could remember everyone who helped me along the way. I sincerely apologize if I forgot to mention anyone in particular. This "blook" is the product of my interactions with a number of people. It was not possible without their input or their influence. I am deeply indebted to every individual I have personally met for shaping who I am. I realize that there is no way to acknowledge EVERYONE. Hopefully this "blanket thank you" will suffice. If you are actually reading this, then I probably know you or I will meet you sometime…so here's a sincere "THANKS" from me to you.

# Table of Contents

# FOREWORD
*Paulette Cebulski PT PhD*

B rain tumors or other potentially catastrophic diagnoses are not the type of diagnoses any of us want to hear. It is no less stressful news if one is old or young, a non-medical person or a health care professional, a usually optimistic person or a pessimistic one, or for any other type of dichotomous descriptions of persons. It is still not the type of news any of us wants to hear. However, how each of us looks at and deals with these types of diagnoses does depend on our age and life space, our outlook on life, be it a glass half full or half empty, and our own frame of reference of understanding the human body, medical terminology and the various possible interventions.

This book, written by Eric Galvez, DPT CSCS, describes the journey of a young health professional who received life-altering news. It chronicles the day-by-day medical experiences, physical and emotional changes and adjustments, and the myriad of psycho-social aspects related to a potentially very devastating diagnosis. The book, written by a physical therapist from the reverse role now as a patient, is intended for rehabilitation education students and for younger active rehabilitation patients. It is written in a conversational and contemporary way consistent with the customs of these groups. However, it also lends great insight into the physical and emotional stages of diagnosis through recovery that could be read by all health care professionals, novice or experienced, and patients and their families, old or young, dealing with these life changing events.

So who is Eric Galvez and why has he asked me to write the foreword to this book? Eric will tell you who he is and the life stage that he is in through each page that he has written in this book. Through his skillful writing, you will quickly visualize him in your mind's eye and feel that you know him well. Through his family and friends' accounts in this book and their observations of his life-altering challenges, you will also get to know Eric. My knowledge of Eric is both a professional and personal one. As a former faculty member and the Director of the Physical Therapy Department at the University of Michigan-Flint where Eric received his Doctor of Physical Therapy degree, I grew to know and admire Eric while he was a student in our program and have maintained a professional and personal relationship with him since his graduation. Eric was a serious student academically who worked hard. But he was not so serious that he did not know how to have fun. He can tell you most of those stories better than I can. But one that he hasn't told you in this book is the lost bet to his Ohio State University (OSU) buddy over the University of Michigan loss to OSU. Eric dutifully donned a pink bunny suit (as in rabbit not a Playboy bunny) and sang "Mr. Sandman" with two of the faculty dressed as tough Harley-Davison bikers at the annual student talent show. He was a sight to behold, but the message was even more profound. Eric knew how to take what others would consider defeat and turn lemons into lemonade. This is the Eric that writes his story. Even in the worst of times and during the toughest days, Eric can find something positive and oftentimes something humorous to keep his spirits up. Wouldn't that be great if we all had this trait?

Through this book I believe Eric will touch and move patients and their families. His down-to-earth approach and "from the heart" way of expressing himself will quickly connect the reader, especially the young adult reader, with his thinking. His positive approach to looking at even the most devastating stages of his recovery and the most challenging of goals can serve as a motivational boost for those in need. His concrete suggestions for patients and their families from lessons he learned as a result of his experience are invaluable for others as they travel their road to recovery.

Students in rehabilitation studies are often given assignments to role-play a disability for a day or a weekend and then reflect on their experiences. Or they may be assigned readings or viewings of videotapes or CDs of persons with disabilities. Often persons with disabilities are brought into classroom to lecture on a topic. All of these serve to aid the student in understanding a little more about the stages of recovery and adjustment to disability. This book and Eric's chronicled journey, told in his vernacular are an outstanding way for students close to his age to better identify with the story than perhaps a more formal presentation. Being a former rehabilitation student himself, he shares insights about recovery that others cannot appreciate. He has viewed and shared his experience of recovery not only as a physical therapist but also as young adult, a son, a brother, a friend, and an all-around great person. The conversational style of writing and the journal entries interspersed with additional reflections and suggestions will lead the reader to read on and on. I believe you will get to know Eric as those of us who have had a small contribution to this book know him. You will be enriched by his account no matter what vantage point you are coming from. It is with this hope that I encourage you to read on…to get to know the Eric Galvez we all know.

Paulette Cebulski, PT, PhD

# Introduction

*Eric Anthony Galvez DPT CSCS*

E very patient has a story. This is mine. In September 2005 I was diagnosed with a non-malignant brain tumor the size of a golf ball on my brainstem and cerebellum. In a month I had brain surgery to have it removed. I also had radiation therapy and a lengthy dose of outpatient physical and occupational therapy. Like most young people, I thought I was invincible. I found out the hard way I'm not. I'm very lucky.

I'm also a walking contradiction. I usually don't read, but here I am writing a book. I'm a "jock," but I've always liked to write. I am a second-generation Filipino-American. My parents were born and raised in the Philippines, but I was born and raised in the US so I am very "Americanized." I'm a physical therapist, but for over a year I was a patient. I somehow ended up in a very strange predicament. As a physical therapist, it's my job to help people regain their function in everyday life. Now, I would be on the receiving end of this relationship. What was even more strange was the fact that the people I used to work side-by-side with were now working with me as a patient. I graduated from Physical Therapy school in Dec 2003. I worked for 6 months in the acute care setting seeing post-surgical patients. I then worked for a year in an outpatient orthopedics clinic seeing patient with back, neck, shoulder or leg pain. After my brain surgery I was left with no coordination, double vision, an extremely weak voice, and the inability to walk. I hoped that this would all be a temporary inconvenience. My cognition and will were 100% normal when I got home, but since I was not perceived by other people as "normal," I got some peculiar responses from people. This is my journey through life as a person with physical impairments.

This book was written for rehab education students and for younger active rehab patients. It is meant to give students an idea of what a patient goes through. It's also meant to give hope to patients going through the rehab process. The book is titled *Reversal: When a Therapist Becomes a Patient* obviously because I'm a physical therapist who became a patient. The title also has a hidden meaning. In high school I was a state champion in wrestling. I would score a lot of my points off of reversals. A reversal is a scoring move where initially your opponent is in control of you. You get points for a reversal when you turn the tables and take control of your opponent. As a patient, one of the hardest things I had to deal with was the loss of control. Everyone around me wanted to be "helpful," especially the people closest to me. Of course I needed help early on, but as I got stronger I felt I could still do many of the things I used to do (not exactly the same way). I felt like I needed people standing beside me more than I needed them standing behind me. It was a struggle getting my sense of control back. There was no way I was going let a damned brain tumor control my life.

The book is a compilation of my personal journal entries/blogs for my friends and family. Most people have blogs to express their opinions about certain topics: political, pop culture, or whatever. All my friends in San Diego have blogs. In fact, one of my friends wrote a book about blogging, *The Rough Guide to Blogging* by Jonathan Yang. I'm sure that if you think of a topic, there is a blog on the internet somewhere dedicated to it. I started it when I moved to San Diego as a way for my friends and family to "keep up" with me.

One afternoon, I was lying in my hospital bed on the rehab unit staring at the ceiling and I had an epiphany. I should share my experiences with students and young patients. I remember how boring the books we read in school were. I remember thinking, "School prepared me for the potential physical challenges I would be up against, but I wish I knew what to expect as a patient. Hmmm... I could write a book! Yeah! Why not, I'll have plenty of time on my hands." I think I told a few people of my grand plan, but they probably laughed it off. The idea got more concrete the longer the rehab process lasted.

Music has always been a large part of my life. I'm always listening to something whenever I'm reading, writing, or studying. There's always a song that captures a moment. Many of the chapters have the names of songs that correspond to the different phases/aspects of my rehab process. The first chapter is entitled *Wake Me Up, When September Ends*. It basically describes how I found out about the tumor, the warning signs, and how I dealt with the scary fact that I had a huge tumor in my head. At the time, I seriously didn't know if I was gonna be alive to see my 31st birthday. The second chapter is entitled *The Final Countdown*. It documents my emotions the month before my surgery and it is my tribute to DEEEEE-TROOOIT BAS-KET-BALL. It was the theme song for the World Champion "Bad Boys" from '89 and '90. The third chapter is called *You Got Another Thing Coming*. It describes my experiences in the intensive care unit, ICU, based on the accounts of the people around me. The fourth chapter, *Livin' on a Prayer*, details my experiences on the rehab unit of the hospital. *Time After Time* is a chapter that describes my fears and experiences with radiation therapy. *Ready or Not* portrays my experiences at home for the first time and my first few months of outpatient therapy. *Don't Stop Believin'* depicts my frustrations with the slow rehab process, my progress in outpatient therapy, and how I coped with my situation. *Back in Black* describes my difficulties and emotions with returning to work. *Best of You* is the chapter that is dedicated to the beginning of 2007 for me. I set some lofty goals and actually got the first edition of this book published. *Rollin'* explores my time focusing on my own rehabilitation with the ultimate goal of returning to the beach to go surfing again. *Stronger* is a chapter that is a peak at the new path I have found in writing and advocacy. *Mr. Brightside* is a chapter that ties updates my progress in rehabilitation, advocacy, and personal goals. It ends opened-ended on purpose to leave the message that the readers are in control of their own destinies. *Photograph* is the title of the pictures section. *Stand by Me* is a song title that captures how I felt about the people closest to me. The chapter describes my relationships with my family, friends, and co-workers throughout the rehab process. I really felt like I needed more people standing beside me than I needed "cheerleaders" standing behind me. *Taking Care of Business* is a song I heard in an office supply store commercial. I decided to use it to title the chapter that involves logistical issues like disability insurance, health insurance, and leave of absence from work. *Learn Yourself* is the title of the chapter dedicated to the life lessons I've learned and used along the way. *Ch-Check It Out* is a song that I used to for a chapter dedicated to "useful resources" for brain tumor patients. *Without Me* is a song I used to title my official biography in the appendix.

The common denominators for a successful rehab process are a positive attitude, a good sense of humor, and a strong support system. I'm very lucky to have a strong group of people that love me. I've dedicated a large portion of the book to my friends and family. I don't think I could have done this by myself. I asked a few people close to me to contribute essays to the book because I thought they could offer a unique perspective on this surprising and extraordinary situation. Their voices were very important because they would be the people I would interact with throughout this strange ordeal.

I asked them to write short essays about their experiences and to title their essays after popular songs to keep with the spirit of the book. I jokingly called this group of people *"the Collective"* like the Borg from *Star Trek* because we shared all of our writing with each other and they were my confidants /counsel during this project. They always knew what I was doing and how I was feeling. First off, I asked my favorite professor from Physical Therapy school, Paulette Cebulski, to write the foreward.

Oliver Galvez, my brother, called his essay *Family Business*. My dad, Jose Galvez, used the song *High Hopes*. My mom, Teresita Galvez, used the song *I'll Be There*. My friends, Mason Tassiviri, Lilly Ghahremani, Christopher Lum, Christopher Thompson DPT, Alvin Borlaza, and Rosalia Machi Arellano MSPT titled their essays: *Ain't No Mountain High Enough* , *True Colors* , *Jesus Walks* , *Believe, Higher,* and *Three Little Birds* respectively. Dan Debeliso, my friend, physical therapist, and former co-worker, titled his essay *Long Road*. Stacey Nelson, my friend and occupational therapist, titled her essay *Learning to Live Again*. Tony Pablo, my friend and occupational therapist titled his essay *KickStart My Heart*. These essays take into account their perspectives on my rehab process because an intimidating diagnosis affects more people than just the patient.

It is my hope that this book elicits an emotion from you. Be it laughter, disgust, or pride. I hope you can somehow relate to my situation. What would you do if you were in my shoes? I promise this won't be your average patient-written book: look out for corny jokes and random pop culture references. For terms that are difficult to understand, refer to the glossary in the appendix section. One afternoon I was listening to my iPod and I thought "I like all these titles/songs. Wouldn't it be cool if there was a book soundtrack?" With a little creativity, I was able to think of a way to make it happen. The book soundtrack is available on iTunes as an iMix. Please visit the web site www.ericgalvezdpt.com for details. I'm not a writer nor will I claim to be one. I published the book because there was a need for something like this. Hopefully it inspires you to do something. Please bear with me through the inadequacies of this book. Enjoy!!!

# Part I:
# My Story

# Wake Me Up When September Ends

Summer has come and passed
The innocent can never last
Wake me up when September ends

**-Green Day**, *American Idiot* 2004

I'm just like you. If you don't think so, then maybe I remind you of your brother, your son, your cousin, your boyfriend, your husband, or maybe even a friend or co-worker of yours. I'm just a regular guy. I like watching football, playing sports, and going to the bar. I had nothing to worry about except changing my fantasy football lineup every Saturday night and deciding what to wear every morning.

Every patient has a story. This is mine. I'm a 30-year-old physical therapist and a very active guy. I'm in the prime of my life. I've never been sick before. I have always been the kind of guy who pushes his physical limits. I learned how to swim just so I could go surfing and do triathlons. I completed 2 sprint triathlons and a half marathon a few months before the surgery. Like many other single men, I moved to the West coast from the Midwest (Michigan) in the hopes of finding a sweet job, an active lifestyle, and a nice girl.

Nothing could have prepared me for the news I was about to receive. Brain cancer/tumors are pretty rare when compared to other types of cancer. In Sept. 2005, I found out that I had a huge brain tumor, a meningioma the size of a golf ball, on the tentorial membrane at the base of my brain between my brain stem and my cerebellum. The brainstem controls a lot of the basic/unconscious bodily functions like heart rate, breathing, balance, and facial/tongue movements. The cerebellum controls balance, coordination, and fine motor skills.

After a little research I found out that according to the American Cancer Society, 2% of all cancer related deaths were attributed to brain cancer. Males have a 0.66% lifetime risk of being diagnosed with a primary malignant brain tumor and a 0.50% chance of dying from a brain tumor. But men are at risk none the less, I never thought it could happen to me. It did. I'm fairly young and in the prime of my life, but I knew what to look out for! According to a study done by the American Cancer Society conducted between 1992-1997, meningiomas are the most common type of primary brain tumors at 27.4%. Emedicine.com stated that meningiomas affect mainly elderly African-American women. The last time I checked, I am none of the above. (I'm a 30-year-old active Filipino-American guy so I obviously don't fall into that category.)

How I overlooked the red flags, I don't know. Hopefully my story will teach you something about identifying the red flags for brain tumors and how to prepare yourself when expecting bad news from health care professionals.

**There are 5 symptoms that could be diagnostic of a brain tumor:**

1. **Headache**
2. **Dizziness**
3. **Nausea**
4. **Facial/ tongue numbness –frequently biting your tongue or lip/cheek**
5. **Loss of appetite**

I had all those signs, but for some reason I ignored them. I learned all about this stuff in physical therapy school. What I didn't realize is that all those symptoms don't necessarily occur at the same time. One day it was the headaches, the next day it was the nausea. At the time I was biting my tongue and lip/cheek pretty frequently. In hindsight I probably couldn't feel them when I was chewing food. Lesson number one: tell the doctor everything.

**Lessons I've learned if expecting bad news**

1. *Tell the doctor everything* – the little "symptoms" might add up to something serious. Maybe you can catch something early before it's too late.

2. *Do your homework*- knowing about your potential condition is half the battle. The internet is a great resource. Websites like www.emedicine.com and www.webmd.com are great resources for the common man for general information. For more detailed research check out www.pubmed.com.

3. *Write down a list of questions for your doctor*- great to do when researching.

4. *Bring at least one other calm person with you to the doctor's office to take notes* - in case you miss anything. You might need another level head on your side.

5. *Don't bring anyone with you who might get too emotional* – (choose your friends/ family members wisely.) The news will be hard enough for you to take. You don't want to have to worry about taking care of anyone else.

Initially I thought the dizziness was due to water in my ear causing an ear infection because I had just starting doing more swimming and surfing. I even had my co-workers look at it to rule out a vestibular problem. I was shocked when I found out it was more serious! You never think it could happen to you. All the warning signs I learned about from school were there. I didn't expect the worst case scenario. I knew something was wrong, but part of me didn't want to definitively find out what was wrong with me. Stupid, I know, but I think that was the reason I was scared to go to the doctor. The following are journal entries/blogs for my friends and family while I was experiencing the symptoms. This is my journey towards discovering I had a tumor and how I dealt with it. Hopefully you can learn how to spot those signs.

Thursday, July 07, 2005

Oh nooooo, I think I have an ear infection. Noticed it a couple of weeks ago, but it's been really flared up over the past few days. I get really dizzy when I swim, run, or do any activity with quick changes of direction. I feel really clumsy after running, swimming, etc. Walking into walls, furniture, people. Damn it... will need to take a week off of swimming and surfing. Guess I gotta start lifting again at least for a little while. I have right beating nystagmus with superior right lateral gaze (looking up and to the right.) Resolves in 30 seconds, but dude it's annoying! I had my co-worker take a look at it to rule out a vestibular problem, she knew exactly how to flare it up. Something is up. I have an appointment with my PCP in 2 weeks, but I think I'll be going to urgent care tomorrow morning just to get this taken care of before I go to Vegas. I hate managed care!

Monday, July 18, 2005

I've been really feeling like crap lately. This dizziness thing is getting really annoying. I haven't run/swum/biked in like 3 weeks. I'm bumping into things. And I have almost no appetite now. Something is wrong. Went to the ENT last week, saw a PA... I guess they just want to wait and see how things go with the Vestibular PT. This is too frustrating. Part of me wants to trust that we are taking the right course of action, but part of me is starting to get a little worried. Maybe it is all down hill after you hit 30.

Tuesday, July 26, 2005

OK, I'm finally starting to feel normal again. The dizziness is getting better and my appetite has returned. I finally had a productive workout this evening.

Sunday, September 11, 2005

I've been having intermittent episodes of dizziness for the past 2-3 months. Things have gotten worse over the last month. I started getting headaches and also noticed a little numbness in the left side of my face. Just last week I started waking up nauseated and vomited a few times. I finally got in to see a doctor last Friday. I was not exactly sure what I was expecting to hear, but deep down I felt like something was just not right.

When I got back to work from the doctor's office I received a message saying that the doctor wanted me to go in later that evening for an urgent MRI at the hospital on my head and neck. I thought, hmmm that's a little weird.

When I got to the hospital, the receptionist said they usually don't do outpatient MRIs at that particular location. So my first thought is either my doc pulled some strings, or something was up. To go from a little dizziness to having an MRI of your head/neck is a pretty big deal. So I was starting to freak out a little bit. So what do I do… sit down kill the time with an old US magazine. Really trivial stuff, but anything to take my mind off what I'm getting tested for. (Jessica Alba has definitely solidified #1 in my "Top 10.") Anyways, the MRI is a huge machine. Basically, you lay down on a conveyor belt then they slide you in. My heart was racing because I've never had anything wrong with me. No broken bones, a concussion here and there, but nothing major.

The test took about one hour. Dude, that's a long time to just lay there and think about stuff. I thought about some pretty random things. Some serious and some not so serious… like do I start Moulds/Jenkins/Calico in my keeper league. I guess I'll be skipping happy hour tonight… that new Kanye song is pretty catchy… Basically stuff to try to keep my mind from scary thoughts. Anyways, the test itself didn't hurt at all. Other than the anxiety, the MRI was not too bad.

So on Saturday morning, I woke up early and tried to put my mind at ease. I started creating playlists on my iTunes. Later a buddy came over, and we headed out to the bar to watch some college football. Anyways, when I got home I noticed a message on the answering machine from my doctor. I made myself a sandwich and then called him. I thought it was a little weird to get a call from the doctor himself. Then he dropped a ton of bricks on me.

He told me he's got some bad news. They found a large mass/tumor on my tentorial membrane at the base of my brain which was applying pressure to all sorts of structures close to my cerebellum and brainstem. He said he didn't think it was malignant or cancerous, but I should see a neurosurgeon for a surgical consult.

Whoa. Whoa. Whoa. Hold on, just a few weeks ago I finished a ½ marathon. I don't do drugs. I'm eating healthier. Sure I drink a little, but for the most part I'm in the prime of my life. I can't be sick.... There is so much more I need to do. Like buying a condo, surfing, the triathlons, moving up the ladder at work, wife, kids… this can't be happening. DAMN IT!

I calmed down by taking some slow deep breaths. The first call I made was to my parents back in the Midwest. I can't even begin to let you know how difficult that was. They took it a lot better than I did. Their calmness definitely made things easier and helped to settle me down. If I stay unemotional, I found that I'm fine when I talk about it. But when people break down in front of me, that's when the kinks in my armor show.


Thursday, September 15, 2005

I got my MRI films and reports today and the official term is "large tentoral-based meningioma." It looks huge. It's amazing how the brain can compensate to such a huge foreign object. I was fine looking at the MRI, but when I showed it to my non-medical friends, I freaked out a little. Just the expressions of fear on their faces made me scared. When I talk to anyone outside of the medical field and I sense any fear in them, it magnifies in me. My emotional state is usually reflective of the people I'm hanging out with.

Before I met with the neurosurgeon, I typed up a list of questions. I had one copy for the doctor and one for my designated note taker. Anyways, I designated my lawyer friend as my note taker. I'm so happy physical therapy school prepared me for this and I was able to play "big words" with the doc. Here are the general questions I had for the neurosurgeon.

**General questions for the doctor:**

1. **What is the prognosis?**
2. **What specific procedures can be done to take this thing out?**
3. **How common is this tumor?**
4. **How did it grow so big? How long do you think it's been there?**
5. **How long is the rehab? What kind of lingering effects should I expect? Timelines?**
6. **Is there a chance for relapse? Is there anything I can do to prevent it from happening again?**
7. **What caused the tumor/where did it come from?**
8. **Am I now at risk for new tumors to pop up?**
9. **When can a procedure be scheduled?**

Whoa… I'm gonna have brain surgery. I always though my first surgery would happen years from now and would be an orthopedic knee or back surgery, not brain surgery and not so soon. In most cases a meningioma isn't malignant and isn't going to directly kill you! That was a huge weight off my shoulders! The location of the tumor scared me the most. The brain stem is one of the most important structures in the body. It controls basic unconscious body functions like heart rate, breathing, and vision to name a few!

Tuesday, September 20, 2005

Whew, this week is a little better. Actually I have to get an angiogram done tomorrow. An angiogram is needed to look at the vasculature or blood supply to the brain. Basically they thread a catheter from my femoral artery in my groin all the way through my heart to the blood vessels in my head. Should take about 1 hour but I'm on bed rest the whole day. Then I see the neurosurgeon again on Thursday. Then the following week I have an appointment with a surgical ENT (Ear, Nose, and Throat doctor). Actually next week I go on medical leave. Who knows how long I'm gonna be out... OK, I'm a little nervous now. I've never called in sick for anything. Weird. Hopefully this is a good idea. I might be imagining things, but I feel like there is more pressure on the left side of my head now... Luckily I see an MD tomorrow and on Thursday.

I'm still in awe of all of this. I'm definitely calling on all my life experiences to deal with all this stuff. I still have no appetite. It's so weird because I'm usually the first to jump at free food, but I seriously have to force myself to eat. So strange. Nothing tastes good and nothing satisfies me.

In a weird way, I'm glad this happened to me and none of my friends/family. I feel like I'm extremely prepared for this. My active lifestyle will prepare me for the physical challenges of rehab. PT school has given me the knowledge base/confidence in the medical profession. I worked for a year as a phlebotomist so the sight of blood doesn't scare me. My surgery will be at the hospital where I used to work so I will know most of the nursing/rehab staff taking care of me. And most of all, my network of friends and family seems to know a lot about these procedures and which doctors are the best surgeons. GO TEAM GALVEZ!!! hahaha!!!!

It's just weird that this happened. Trust me, I've thought about all the risk factors: familial history, aspartane (nutrasweet), cell phone use? I could probably make some sort of loose connection to any of these risk factors but I still don't see how/why something like this happens. I'm not perfect, but I've always tried to do the right thing. It's not fair, but sometimes there is nothing you can do. Things just happen. Then you really see what you're made of. This really puts a lot of things in perspective. For me, family comes first but how do you prioritize your life after that? This has really made me realize how much my family means to me. I can only imagine how much stress they must be going through. I'm not even that nervous yet. It's crazy. I feel like this is all just a bad dream. I'm ready to wake up now! I'll be really glad when my parents get out here just so I know they are OK because honestly I'm fine right now. What is wrong with me? I can't wait to come home for Christmas, so I can see everyone else and give them a big hug!

Wednesday, September 21, 2005

I just had my angiogram: the L meningohypophyseal trunk and the left superior cerebellar arteries are the main blood supply for the tumor. I've been feeling worse lately so I had a stat CT scan yesterday. I was prepared to get admitted for a shunt placement, but apparently it's still not that bad yet. I just wanna get this thing out! I MUST PROTECT THIS HOUSE!!! hee hee hee. I'm more tired than anything right now. Just exhausted. This has been a lot to absorb in the past 2 weeks. My dad just got out here last night so I'll have 24-hour supervision. I kinda feel like I'm "grounded" or "expelled." Can't go to work. Can't go surfing. Can't go to the gym. Gotta lay low. hahaha.... Actually, I've never gotten expelled before, but I'm guessing this is what it would feel like.

Tuesday, September 27, 2005

I won't lie. I feel like shit. I'm so tired, the headaches are there all the time, and the vomiting started again. I see the neurosurgeon tomorrow morning and the ENT on Thursday. I can't wait to get this out so I can feel better again. My dad is cooking for me and driving me around. Too bad I'm not hungry. Anyways, I'm hanging in there. I'd much rather be at work. Will keep you guys updated once I see the ENT. Hopefully I'll have surgery date by then... I have a feeling I'm gonna need to consult with both the ENT and neurosurgeon again... Whoa, how many people our age can say they have an ENT and a neurosurgeon? Weird...

Thursday, September 29, 2005

Well, things have finally taken a little turn for the better. I went to see the neurosurgeon yesterday because like I said, the nausea/vomiting and headaches have been getting worse over the past week. I felt horrible. So anyways the neurosurgeon prescribed me some steroids to help control the edema. So I took some prednisone yesterday... this morning was the first morning in about 2 weeks that I woke up without a headache! Definitely helping to control the swelling, but the tumor is still there. The dizziness is still there, but no HA (headaches) or nausea! Yes!!!! I actually stopped by work yesterday just to say "hi." Actually I went in to finish up some paperwork and to get out of the house. It hasn't even been a week yet, but I'm already getting cabin fever. It was so good seeing everyone, and it feels really good knowing that people are in your corner!

Today was actually a pretty good day. Ran some errands with my pops. Took the roof rack off my car. So sad... My car looks so naked. I'll put it back on after the surgery and when I'm ready to go surfing/biking again... Oooooh getting back in the water is gonna feel soooo good!! But today I finally got some more definite answers to my questions.

I guess in terms of the procedure, they will go behind the left ear and cut through the skull. Next they will need to retract part of the brain (temporal lobe) to access the tumor. And then they go in with a scope that will chop up and suck up the tumor with hopefully minimal damage to the nerves and arteries in that area. This kinda messes my plan for keeping it in a jar and naming it "Amani Toomer." Hee hee. At least it will be out! They might need to put a lumbar shunt in to control the pressure of the CSF (cerebrospinal fluid)... so basically there is potential for another huge hole in my body (somewhere in the low back... aw man!!!) I'm telling you I've had so many needles and blood draws recently that they don't even phase me anymore.

The surgery should take about 4 hours because it's pretty big, but it really depends on the consistency of the tumor. (In actuality it took over 12 hours.) If it is stuck on a nerve or artery it will definitely make things more complicated. Gulp... If not, then it could be quicker. Apparently once the size of the tumor starts to decrease, the brain reoccupies the empty space and hopefully makes it easier to remove. I think that this applies for tumors on the perimeter of the cranium, not underneath around the brainstem… The nerves at risk are the trigeminal nerve, the facial nerve, and the auditory nerve. The ENT believes the major arteries aren't at risk, but again it depends if the tumor is stuck to the artery. The carotids are pretty vital in terms of supplying blood to the brain. The ENT also believes that if things go well… I shouldn't need to get admitted to rehab and will probably need outpatient rehab for Bell's palsy (facial paralysis) like symptoms and hearing loss, which worse-case scenario could take a few months or a full year to recover. So that news is pretty good, but there is still that unknown element that could pop up and make things "difficult." Damn, there are so many "ifs"… argh!!! And it looks as if the surgery date will be in the 3rd week of October. I wish it could be sooner though. I just want this thing out! At least for now the headaches and the nausea are better controlled. Hopefully I'll have an actual date tomorrow when I call the neurosurgeon. If not, I should have a solid date by Tuesday! The waiting is what sucks the most!!! Now we know what needs to be done, how to do it, so LET'S DO THIS!!! Like I mentioned before, I think things are finally starting to turn the corner. Let's hope that this thing will cooperate and not stick to anything. But the main thing is right now no major headaches or vomiting!!! Let's hope this lasts till my surgery date. Whenever that may be…

After I found out about the tumor I figured I'd be out only a few months and I would be back at work treating patients again. Man, I was way off!!! I would be in the intensive care unit for 8 days and in the hospital for 5 weeks. Outpatient rehab would last for over a year! The location and size of the tumor were the scariest things to deal with. Now it's just a waiting game and the most terrifying thing I've ever had to deal with… my own mortality.

# The Final Countdown

I guess there is no one to blame
We're leaving ground
Will things ever be the same again?
It's the Final Countdown...

**-Europe**, *The Final Countdown* 1986

I had to wait a month before my surgery. I didn't know anyone that had the same problem/diagnosis as I had. It was the scariest thing I've had to deal with so far in life. I really didn't know how things were gonna turn out. Since the tumor was so close to the brainstem, there was the risk that something serious could go wrong and I could die or be on a ventilator for the rest of my life. Those were worst case scenarios. I kept telling myself that it's out of my hands now and to just enjoy the company of my family and friends.

I've never had surgery or been to the hospital on behalf of myself or my parents. Actually I take that back, I went to the hospital to get an MRI of my head done a month before my surgery. It was kinda intimidating going in there alone. I didn't want to go by myself again, so who do I bring with me for brain surgery? My parents and my aunt. My friends offered to be there but I wanted to be with my family. Since I don't have my own family (wife/kids) yet, I figured they will do. I wouldn't want to put my friends or a girlfriend through the hell my parents went through.

I guess we were told the night before that the surgery would last all day. What!!! Is that humanly possible? I'm sure they have to take bathroom breaks at some point! I was in the operating room for over 12 hours. I went down to the OR for anesthesia at 6:30 AM. My parents didn't see me until 9PM. I guess they were freaking out/stressing out. They didn't hear anything from the doctors or nurses for a while. They were in the dark about where I was and if I was doing OK. I can't even imagine the stress involved with that ordeal. They didn't hear anything about how the surgery was going, if I was OK, or even if the surgery was over. Dude, I can't even imagine waiting under those circumstances for news about a child or even a loved one.

I had to go on state disability and take an official leave of absence from work from 9/21/05 to 9/21/06. After an angiogram to look at the vasculature or blood supply around my brain I felt horrible. I was unable to function at work. My dad had just retired so he actually flew out to San Diego from Michigan to drive me to appointments and help me out at home. (He would be with me for over a year!) Before the surgery, I was feeling pretty sick. I was in pretty bad shape. Dizziness and vomiting were part of my daily routine. The weeks leading up to my surgery were filled with uncertainty and fear of the unknown. I used this time to reflect on everything I had accomplished. I usually don't think about the "meaning of life" or other existential concepts, but a brush with your mortality brings those ideas to the surface. The following are journal entries/blogs for my friends and family.

Tuesday, October 04, 2005

It's the Final Countdown… OK, here is the tentative date: October 25th! Damn. That's 3 weeks away. Seems like a long time to wait. I'm calling again in the morning to see if I can get in any sooner. I just got approval from my insurance for a "Craniotomy for tumor removal."

Saturday, October 08, 2005

Argh…. I feel horrible again. Looks like the date is in stone. October 25th is the day. Dude, I really feel like crap now. Yesterday went to the beach and spent a few hours there reading (don't laugh) *Harry Potter and the Half Blood Prince*. The headaches are back and I can definitely feel pressure behind my L eye. The numbness is now around my left eye. The throwing up is better controlled, but still occasionally happens. I think it might be time to go back on the steroids to control the swelling.

Maybe it's the tumor or maybe it's the way the Michigan offense is playing right now.

Thursday, October 13, 2005

OK, I'm better now. That prednisone stuff (a steroid) works pretty well. It's supposed help with my appetite too, but so far I haven't noticed a huge difference. I am eating though, so that's good. Hmmm… Anyways, I'm still pretty bored. I've gone to the beach a few times to read. I'm still laughing at myself for reading *Harry Potter and the Half Blood Prince*. It's got me occupied. I was thinking to myself, this isn't so bad. I've got my dad out here to hang out with, drive me around, and to cook for me. I'm in a beautiful place that's sunny and 70 degrees most of the time, so I can chill at the beach. It's the fall, so there is some sort of football on TV all the time. I can get Fox Sports Detroit with the satellite which equals preseason Pistons, Red Wings, and home town coverage of the Lions/U of M. I have 3 months of all the movie channels (HBO, Showtime, Stars, Cinemax) free for signing up for DirecTv.

Actually I've watched 35 different movies so far. And yes, I have them all documented and rated on a five-point scale on my computer. I'm shooting for 60 before I have to go back to work. Anyways, I find myself watching a lot of the movies from the 80's and 90's that I watched as a latch-key kid during summer vacation. My favorite one so far has got to be *The Karate Kid*. The soundtrack alone is vintage 80's. Dude, there are some classic lines from that movie. There are the obvious ones. "Wax on, Wax off," "Sand the floor," "Paint the fence," etc. … but the other more subtle ones are the ones I enjoy the most. Me and my younger brother used to act out the scene at the end where Daniel assumes the "ready" position, the soundtrack gets really intense, Johnny gets crane kicked in the face, then he grabs his face and crawls off camera on his hands and knees. Too funny. Then with cheesy 80's victory music in the background, Johnny comes back with the trophy for Daniel and he says "You're alright Larusso. You're alright." Conflict Resolved! The smirk on Mr. Miagi's face at the end is classic. Always makes me laugh hahaha… whew. Watch it again, I guarantee you'll laugh now, too. God, I love those cheesy 80's movies.

Anyways, on a side note… I'm not sure if there is any science behind this, but I do notice that after I watch a funny/stupid movie or after a night hanging out with my friends, I do feel a little better. The headaches are less intense. The dizziness doesn't feel as bad. Maybe there is some truth to "laughter is the best medicine."

Monday, October 17, 2005
**WHAT IF….**
… I went to MSU or Purdue for undergrad instead of U of M
… I decided to work in Michigan after PT school
… I decided to join a traditional Greek Fraternity and not Lambda Phi Epsilon
… I never got the chance to join the college a capella group 58 Greene at the University of Michigan
… I decided to go to PT school in California
… I decided to move to LA or Sacramento instead of San Diego
… I didn't get a concussion snowboarding in Tahoe
… I decided to work in a private clinic
… I had my condition 50 years ago
… They don't get everything
… I wake up from surgery and I'm on a vent/respirator
… I wake up from surgery and I can't move the right side of my body
… I don't wake up from surgery
… I said "hi" to the hot girl
… I didn't drink too much
… I had a beer tonight
… I started eating fast food again
… I never fell in love
… I never got my heart broken
… I never got into running/triathlons
… I never learned how to surf or snowboard

... I didn't believe in God

... God has something BIGGER planned for me.

No one knows the definite answers to these questions. All I know is I feel like I've made all the right choices so far and I have no regrets. There are still a lot of things I need to do. Just one more week to wait, then this thing will be out. This thing has really been a test of my faith and my patience. I'm positive I'll come out of this a stronger person, a better friend, and a more understanding therapist. I go in for another CT scan tomorrow then a couple pre-op appointments this week. Surgery is on Tuesday next week. Part of me is relieved the date is getting closer. The other part of me is just NOW starting to get a little nervous. My mom and aunt are flying in next Monday. Wow. This is really happening!

Thursday, October 20, 2005

Looks like the incision is going to be bigger than I initially thought it was going to be... All the way around my ear. I'm told that the hair will grow back, but maybe I'll just keep it shaved all the time now. Yesterday morning I threw up twice. I couldn't keep anything down. Luckily, I had another appointment with the neurosurgeon that afternoon. He took me off of prednisone and is starting me on dexamethasone, another steroid. I've heard some nasty stuff about the side effects. I'm gonna try to stay off the medication as much as I can. But sometimes I really need it.

In case you are wondering what I'm going though, imagine the worst hangover you've ever had... the unsteadiness, the feeling of nausea, and the headache... add a little numbness on your left cheek and tongue and there you have it. Now grant it, I'm not like this all the time, but there are some mornings when the only reason I get out of bed is to rush to the bathroom to throw up. The steroids help immensely, but on the days I'm off of them... yuck. Not pleasant to be around... I have a hard time walking a straight line, but I can do it if I go really slow. Everything moves really slow, not like elderly person slow, but definitely slower than normal. Now would be a good time to race me if you want to win.

I've kinda shifted my focus from movies to reading. Currently on: *Lance Armstrong's It's Not about the Bike, Harry Potter The Half Blood Prince,* and *the Essence of Swiss Ball Training.* Definitely not bored anymore. Thank God I'm not bored. I almost watched the Olivia Newton John roller skating epic *Xanadu* earlier this week! Damn! That definitely has to be my lowest point. When I realized what I was watching, I was like "OK, I need to put an end to this downward spiral!" You can only watch so much TV and that was my breaking point. I also found out I suck at video games. In *Halo* I keep running into walls, in *Madden* I can't pass or play defense, in racing I can't take turns without hitting the wall... I wasted too much time the past few years "playing" outside or going to the gym so I'm a little behind in my gaming skills...

As for my mental state... honestly I think right now I'm more worried about the Foley catheter. You would be, too, if you knew where it goes and how it gets there. (It's basically a tube they stick in your penis that runs to all the way up to your bladder to help with urine excretion.) I've been told that I'll probably be out when they put it in, but I'll wake up with it in me and I'll be awake when they take it out... that's gonna hurt =(

Dude, I'm gonna be buck naked in front of bunch of people. I don't know how I feel about that! I don't like being naked in front of myself, let alone 10-15 strangers! Hopefully I'll at least get some cute nurses to take care of me... My OR time is from 7:30 to 3:30... Jeez, that's got to be enough time to get everything! It seems like a long time to me. I wonder if they take coffee breaks or lunch breaks.

Anyways the reality of brain surgery is finally sinking in. I've had 2 pre-op appointments this week. I guess there is a serious chance that I might lose the hearing in my left ear. Apparently they will cut into the Mastoid and Temporal bones. They are trying to avoid the semi-circular canals if possible, but if they can't access the whole tumor they will need to go through the semicircular canals to get everything. If that happens, there is a 99% chance I lose the hearing in the left ear and I will definitely have more problems with dizziness for a few more months.

Kinda sucks that the initial problem that I was having could be a side effect for the treatment of the tumor. Well, at least I have another ear and I won't be completely deaf. Whoa. This is real, no more talk… this is gonna happen! So on Saturday, I'm going to SeaWorld to take my mind off of things. Sunday will be another day of football. Monday will be my quiet prep day. I guarantee I'll feel like shit DOS (day of surgery), but Wed POD 1(post-op day 1) I should be able to take visitors. Probably not for too long but it will be nice to have visitors. By Thursday I should be much better and able to tolerate more. No crazy bar hopping or anything, but maybe a friendly game of "Cranium.".. har har har.


Monday, October 24, 2005

Looks like I'll get admitted tonight. Just got a call from the hospital. Was supposed to go in at 5AM tomorrow. Slight curveball.

I know a lot of you wish you could be here with me. I'll strike a deal. This is the playlist I'll be listening to tonight on my I-pod. Just play one of the songs and you're there with me.


**Lose Yourself** -Eminem
**Mr. Brightside** - The Killers
**It's So Easy** – Guns N Roses
**Breakout** - Foo Fighters
**Higher Ground** - Red Hot Chili Peppers
**Gold Digger** – Kanye West
**Jesus Walks** – Kanye West
**Ready or Not** –The Fugees
**Superstition** – Stevie Wonder
**In the Air Tonight** – Phil Collins
**A Little Respect** - Erasure (don't laugh)

*The Promise* - When in Rome
*Only You* - Yaz ( I like this song OK!)
*Don't Stop Believing* - JOURNEY!
*Blaze of Glory* - Bon Jovi
*THE FINAL COUNTDOWN* - EUROPE!

The surgery went well. Please see the accounts of my family and friends regarding what happened next. That is where my memory escapes me. At least the dangerous part was over. Now it's time to recover in the ICU (Intensive Care Unit). I was there a lot longer than I expected!

# You Got Another Thing Comin'

If you think I'll sit around as the world goes by
You're thinkin' like a fool cause it's a case of do or die
Out there is a fortune waitin' to be had
You think I'll let it go you're mad
You've got another thing comin'

**-Judas Priest,** *Screaming for Vengeance* 1982

My memory of the ICU is very limited. Most of this chapter was based on the accounts of the people close to me. Initially I thought this was gonna be piece of cake. I thought I would be in and out of the hospital in a couple of weeks. Boy, was I way off! I thought I'd be out of surgery and in the Intensive Care Unit, ICU, for only a day. I ended up in the ICU for 8 days. I also thought I'd be in the hospital a couple of days. Turns out I would be in the hospital for over 5 weeks.

Honestly I don't remember much from the ICU, but I do vaguely recall having my right arm restrained and tied to the table. I was held in the ICU for 8 days due to post-surgical complications. Postoperatively, I spiked a fever of unknown origin. They were thinking it could be an infection in my gall bladder, an infection in the urethra from the Foley, or something else dealing with my stomach or intestines. I guess I also had no sensation around my left cheek and no movement of my left eyelid. I also had a lot of ataxia/tone in the left side of my body. Initially the surgeon said he got 45% of the tumor but later we were told he got 95% of the tumor.

I had so many tubes coming out of me and I was heavily sedated. Thank God I don't remember too much because I was most nervous about the Foley catheter. They usually put in the catheter right before the surgery when you are under anesthesia. Unfortunately, I do remember them taking it out. The nurse showed it to me after she took it out. I remember turning my head away quickly so I wouldn't see the length of the tubing or any blood left on it.

I was in really bad shape. I couldn't sit up straight. The ataxia in my left arm and leg was horrible. My arm and leg would flail all over the place if I tried to voluntarily move them. I had just been extubated so my voice was really weak and I had a hard time swallowing. I would have to wear a neck brace to keep my head up and an eye patch because I couldn't blink my left eye..

I guess the nurses and many of my co-workers were really helpful to my family for which I'll forever be grateful. Supposedly I was a handful in the ICU. Somehow I got my hands on my cell phone and I called my Mom at 2 in the morning and asked her to pick me up and take me home. She was tough and held her ground. I imagine it takes a lot to say NO to your eldest son, but I must have really wanted out of there. Evidently, I also tried getting up out of bed a couple of times which got my right hand restrained and tied to the bed. I have no recollection of these events at all. When I heard this I was shocked! I'm usually pretty reserved and laid back.

At least the dangerous and scary part was over. I was still mentally out of it. I barely knew where I was and the current date. I was also on seizure precautions, but I don't recall having a seizure. I still had to figure what I could and couldn't do. It always cracks me up in movies how the hero goes to the hospital and leaves within a few hours. Too bad it doesn't work like that. They totally skip the whole rehab process. Up next for me, the hard part... the start of rehabilitation in the hospital.

# Livin' on a Prayer

Whooah, were half way there
Livin' on a prayer
Take my hand and well make it - I swear
Livin 'on a prayer

**-Bon Jovi**, *Slippery When Wet* 1986

After the ICU I got transferred to another floor. I was there for a few days, then I got transferred to the rehab unit. I vaguely recall that intermediate floor. I remember my uncle and aunt came to visit me from Toronto. I also remember really wanting a "Big Mac." I used to be a huge junk food addict before the surgery. I had just started cutting down on my junk food intake the summer before the surgery. I also remember watching *Star Wars Episode III, Revenge of the Sith* on a laptop with a buddy when it first came out on DVD in my hospital room. I'm a huge Star Wars dork. In college I sent 2 *"Kellogg's Fruit Loops"* Proofs of Purchase for a free mail order Special Edition Storm Trooper Han Solo action figure with removable helmet.

Anyways, to qualify for rehab you have to be able to tolerate 3 hours of therapy a day. It was also the place where I would come out of my post-surgical fog. I remember when I first got transferred to rehab, there were concerns about not having a bowel movement in 8 days. I remember that vividly because if I didn't have a BM I would be given a suppository.

I was really determined to avoid that suppository. When you have a suppository, they stick a small (I hoped it was small, I refused to look at it) tablet up your butt. So the first thing I thought of was eating a burrito. They always "worked" before. I had one of my physical therapy aide friends grab me a California burrito (a carne asada burrito packed with marinated meat, cheese, guacamole, salsa, and get this… French fries) from a local taco shop. Unfortunately, I had swallow precautions. So that would limit my enjoyment of my burrito. Nothing would stop me though. I was gonna have that burrito. I was positive this was gonna work so I could avoid that suppository. The California burrito has never "failed" me before. It had to work…

After praying for a last ditch burrito-eating miracle, I ended up getting the suppository anyways. Not very pleasant. I remember lying on my side facing the wall and being extremely tense. I was pretty scared. I ask a lot of questions when I'm nervous. "Wait, wait, wait… How long does this usually take? Wait, wait, wait… Are you gonna give me any warning before you put it in? Wait, wait, wait… Are you gonna GO on 'three' and then do it, or are you gonna say 'three' and then do it? Wait, wait, wait… How deep in does it have to go?" I pleaded with the nurses to be gentle. They just inserted it, and then it was done. Quick and Easy. I think I was crying with nervous laughter the whole time. Whew. In about 20 minutes things were moving. I've never wanted to take a dump so bad in my entire life! It's funny looking back at that whole ordeal, but I don't want to go through that EVER again!

One of the hardest things for me to get used to was getting naked in front of people. Dude, I don't like being naked in front of myself, let alone a bunch of strangers. The shower was odd. I had to transfer to a special shower chair in the room then get wheeled down to the shower room. In the shower, they would take off layer by layer till you were buck naked. They let you scrub your own groin area, but everything else was fair game. I had to put a plastic bag over my PICC line to prevent water from getting in and potentially causing an infection. It was kind of weird having someone shampoo my head, but at the same time kind of nice. I don't think I'll ever spend big bucks at a fancy salon, but even though I had no hair after cutting it short for the surgery, the scalp messaging felt pretty good. By the end of my time in rehab I had no qualms about getting buck naked in front of the nursing assistants. Drop my pants, no problem… Most of the nursing assistants treated me like their son, which was a good but sometimes annoying thing.

At first I could barely sit up without support. I had severe ataxia in my left arm and leg. I also had to wear an eye patch over my left eye because the left side of my face was paralyzed. A week of inactivity really takes a lot out of you. Sitting in a chair without back support seemed impossible. At first I was drooling a lot and I wanted to get moving more on my own. You must have the normal mobility progression before you can start walking:

1. **Good sitting balance/core stability**
2. **Good static standing balance**
3. **Good dynamic standing balance**
4. **Good leg coordination**

Every morning my Occupational Therapist helped me get ready for my busy day of rehab. I always wondered what they did with patients. Back when I worked acute care I actually did a few co-evaluations on patients with some of the OTs. I've read their notes, but I've never sat in on an OT treatment. I'm not a morning person, so I always made sure that I was awake for at least one hour before they came in. I would always watch the Today show while I waited for them to come. I've always been strangely attracted to Katie Couric. Anyways, the OTs showed me how to put on a shirt and shorts with one hand. I still couldn't stand up by myself, so I had to get dressed laying down or sitting down. It was a lot harder than I thought.

I had a bunch of different OTs in rehab, but they all were excellent. As a PT I always thought the stuff they did with patients was really mundane. I couldn't believe how much we take for granted as able-bodied individuals. Getting dressed in the morning, brushing your teeth, and washing your face seem like routine or automatic tasks, but for someone with physical impairments it's like climbing a mountain. Now, I realize the importance of their work. I have so much respect for them and their work. They were all really easy to talk to as well.

I was not too familiar with speech therapy before the surgery. From my understanding the speech therapists were in charge of my swallowing and reasoning/memory. I guess my voice was really weak and I couldn't swallow anything, based on what people are telling me. I stuffed my face at my first meal. I kept shoveling food into my mouth without chewing or swallowing. In speech therapy we did a lot of attention type activities and facial muscle and tongue exercises. Actually, I am really grateful for all the help they gave me. By the end of my sessions I came to the realization as to what I was saying. I was cracking up because many of the phrases were geared towards an older population. Whenever I was reading some thing really obscure, it totally set me off. My laughter soon spread to the therapist. Those were fun sessions.

I also had one pool therapy session while I was on rehab. I was cracking jokes my first time in the pool. Those little floating devices make a lot bubbles. Me, being the mature healthcare professional, couldn't hold it back. I kept laughing whenever the bubbles came up. All I would have to do was look at the people helping me dead in the eye and everyone would start laughing. I don't know how many times I made myself and everyone around me laugh that afternoon.

While I was in the pool one of the therapists made a comment to the aide helping us about some yellow bathing suit some old lady in the water aerobics class was wearing. We had to share pool time with the water aerobics class. All I heard from their conversation was "yellow in the water" plus we were in the pool with a bunch of elderly people so naturally I assumed someone peed in the water! I guess I really wanted out of the pool at that point. I was cracking the other therapists up about that one.

The most memorable times I had in the hospital were when my friends came to visit. I remember seeing my friends for the first time. I was about to take a shower with the assistance of a nursing aide. All the smack talk came out from my friends. I felt like a normal guy again. Whenever they were there, I didn't feel like a patient. One weekend they brought in pizza. I think I was still on a soft diet, but I didn't care.

I **wanted** a Meat Lover's pizza. All the nurses were keeping a close eye on me. Man, I felt like I had some illegal contraband or something. I even had one of my co-workers tape the U of M-Ohio State game for me, so I could watch it later in the recreation room. Unfortunately I found out the final score before I had a chance to watch it, so I didn't feel like watching it anymore

I never felt alone while I was in the hospital. That was my biggest fear, falling in a rut and getting depressed. My coworkers would come visit me often. It was nice having familiar faces dropping by so often. Knowing the staff where you have surgery has its perks and drawbacks. I got the best treatment, but I also had a lot of visitors. I liked the friendly atmosphere, but it left me with very little privacy.

**Pros and Cons of going through rehab where you work:**
*Pros*
1. **You'll get the best care.**
2. **Your co-workers will be great advocates for you.**
3. **Lots of support.**
4. **You'll be familiar with protocols/policies and procedures.**

*Cons*
1. **So many visitors, very little privacy.**
2. **Your co-workers will see you at your worst.**
3. **It's like you're still going to work.**
4. **Different perceived roles with your co-workers.**

The hardest thing for me to deal with in rehab was knowing what needed to be done to progress, but not being able to do it. I really think it was harder on my family than it was on me because I knew what to look for in terms of progress. I had to explain to my parents every day that things were going well, specifically with weight shifting and balance. They would only look at the big functional goals like walking distance and speed. It was tough trying to tell both my parents to stay patient because I shared their impatience. They were so used to cheering me on as an athlete that I think it was a difficult adjustment for them to make.

My relationship with my co-workers was a little odd at first. Actually I don't remember much from my first days in the ICU, but I'm sure they were there. In rehab, my head was clearing up and I was becoming more aware of my surroundings. We kept things pretty professional whenever someone I knew was working with me. Sure, we would joke around occasionally, but there was mutual respect on both sides. What I really appreciated was my therapist asking me what I wanted to work on at the beginning of each session, while still setting certain objectives each session. I also appreciated the feedback on the identification of my impairments so I could attempt to correct them myself. Sometimes we get so used to telling patients what to do, we forget to tell them why we are doing certain activities.

Setting goals really kept me going. The goals I set for myself helped me to focus on what I needed to do. It really made me feel like I was in charge of my own destiny. One of the biggest things taken away from me was my independence. The sense of control is something every patient should have.

**Things to remember when working with patients**

1. **Check-in periodically - Always ask their opinion on how they feel things are going.**
2. **Involve them in the treatment planning.**
3. **Help them set attainable functional goals.**
4. **Explain why they are doing certain activities.**
5. **Listen to their concerns. Don't forget they spend more time with you than with their docs.**
6. **Remind them that maximum progress is made outside of the therapy sessions through their HEP ( home exercise program).**

People ask me how I dealt with everything. My response to them was every day was different with new challenges. I know this is a cliché, but I seriously had to take it one day at a time. I would wake up every morning and certain things would be a little easier. Each day brought a different challenge. Treating and beating each new challenge individually made the days go by faster. I never let go of the belief that I'm still a regular guy that takes a little longer to do common everyday activities. I'm still a pretty immature guy so I took the time to laugh at myself and all the difficult situations I put myself in.

The whole time in rehab I just wanted to go home and get back to work. Everything I did was geared towards going home. I was halfway there. Once I got home, I figured that I would be one step closer to returning to work and back to normal. I already missed Thanksgiving; I didn't want to miss Christmas, too. The quicker I went home, the quicker I could go back to work and end this nightmare. Little did I know, that was only the beginning. Outpatient rehab and radiation therapy were still waiting for me.

# Time After Time

If you're lost you can look--and you will find me
time after time
If you fall I will catch you--I'll be waiting
time after time

**-Cyndi Lauper,** *She's So Unusual* 1983

I didn't personally know of anyone that had gone through radiation therapy. None of my patients or my parents' friends had ever had it. I knew aunts and parents of friends that have gone through chemo, but this was a totally new and undiscovered experience. I really didn't know what to expect. Someone told me that I should expect a lot of fatigue and to lose some hair where the radiation enters the head. I was going to have a specialized kind of radiation: tomotherapy.

Tomotherapy is a new type of cancer/tumor treatment that combines imaging from a CT scan with delivery of radiation treatments. From my understanding this makes it more accurate than traditional radiation therapy.

This was a very intimidating machine. It looked like a standard MRI machine, but there was so much involved with the setup. They mold a mesh mask of your head, then strap the mask to the table. The mask keeps your head still during the treatment. You don't want to move accidentally and "zap" something other then the tumor! The table then slides into the machine which I dubbed "the Cave." Some people would freak out in the Cave if they're claustrophobic. Before they slide you into the machine, they give you a panic button to press if you freak out. If you freak out, you are then administered sedative medication to calm down.

The tomotherapy radiation sessions had two parts: a scan and a treatment. The total time in there took about 20 minutes. The scan took about 5 minutes. Basically, the scan was performed to make sure everything was lined up. From my understanding the scan pinpointed the areas where the radiation would penetrate. The actual treatment was a little longer. This is when the actual radiation was delivered. I also remember smelling some burning in the middle of each treatment.

I had radiation treatments for 6 weeks, 5 days a week, with PT and OT sessions Monday, Wednesday, and Friday. I made sure that my PT and OT sessions were before my radiation sessions because I was expecting to be fatigued after radiation. When I first heard about this I couldn't believe what lay ahead for me. I just wanted to get back to work. These radiation sessions would definitely slow down my progress.

I was a little scared to go in there the first time because the rest of the patients in the waiting room looked really sick. Nobody was my age. Someone told me not to open my eyes in "the Cave" to prevent getting claustrophobic. My strategy was to shut my eyes and count as high as I could. Each session I promised myself I would not open my eyes till I was done with the treatment. I think I closed my eyes as tight as I could the first few sessions. I really didn't want to "freak out."

I must have been pretty wiped out whenever I went in the Cave because I fell asleep 80% of the time. The nurses were amazed that I could fall asleep so fast in the Cave with all the loud noises. The counting would start to get slow around 350"

I'm not going to lie. It sucked going in everyday. I lost a pretty big patch of hair behind my left ear after about 4 weeks. I was so tired and fatigued after each session. It took me about an hour to regain my energy. I didn't feel comfortable walking so I used the wheelchair at the end of each session. The last two weeks of radiation, every Tuesday and Thursday, I would walk in with the walker but leave in the wheelchair.

Just from talking to people in the waiting room, I learned so much. This is where I learned that every patient has a story and each patient deals with things differently. Nothing is textbook. One guy I would talk to everyday had his own strategy for dealing with the Cave. He always got dropped off for his appointments early. He was a few weeks ahead of me in treatments and his appointments were always right after mine. Anyways, he said that he would count the number of clicks in the machine to stay sane in the Cave. He said he actually had to use the panic button in the machine when he first started his treatments. The counting took his mind off of things. When we first started talking, he thought I was still in high school or college. I guess that's a compliment, but it would always make me mad when I first turned 21.

The nurses were really cool to me. I think I stick out because I'm not a typical radiation patient and I look younger than I really am. I'm the guy that still gets carded every time I go out. Most of the patients in there were my parents age or older, but I felt more connected to them than the regular rehab patients. We were fighting together. I guess the big difference here was the fact that I would see the other radiation patients only when we were coming in/out of appointments. I remember getting nods and "eye-contact high fives" from patients in line or exiting their radiation appointments. I would soon be giving out those non-verbal gestures after a few sessions. We were all "fighting" the effects of that machine. We all had the same side effects.

Honestly, I felt fine for the first four weeks, but when that fifth week rolled around I felt so tired. No nausea, memory loss, or any other side effects... just really sleepy and completely wiped out. I've never felt like that after a tough wrestling or football practice. Very strange.

I had no personal experience with radiation so I had no idea what to expect. After my first radiation session, I was not feeling any effects from the radiation. Around the 4th week I started to feel the effects. The following are journal entries and blogs after I got discharged home. I had just started outpatient physical therapy, occupational therapy, and speech therapy as well as my radiation therapy sessions.

Wednesday, December 14, 2005

Met with the radiologist today and had my 2nd day of outpatient therapy. Looks like I'll be discharged from outpatient speech on Monday.

PT is going well; hopefully I'll be walking more independently in a few weeks so I can get out if this wheelchair. Damn you ataxia!!! I'm trying to type with 2 hands today. Man, so many typos... Anyways the meeting with the radiologist kind of freaked me out. There is a small chance something can go wrong... that means there is still a chance! Based on the location of the tumor remains... the brainstem is still at risk.... Scary.

There is also a chance the tumor might come back. Either everything I've been doing so far will eradicate the tumor, or postpone the return of the tumor/symptoms a few more years. Jeez... what great news. It's the doctor's job to inform me of all possible outcomes, but I wish I was more prepared for this. I keep reminding myself those are worst-case scenarios.

It didn't help that both of my parents looked scared while we waited for the oncologist. The biggest side effects will be severe fatigue and hair loss. I say **"Bring it!"** Fatigue gives me an excuse to eat more, and my hair is short anyways. I think I'll definitely need some prayers now.... I was not as prepared for this doctor visit.

Friday, December 16, 2005

Radiation starts 1/3/06 and will go on for 6-7 weeks. I also got fitted for my radiation mask today. The mask will keep my head from moving during treatments.

Tuesday, January 03, 2006

Today was my first day of radiation therapy and no, I didn't see any radioactive spiders or anything.... Some of you might get that. Anyways, it wasn't as bad as I thought. Took about 20 minutes total. It is a little claustrophobic lying in the Cave and being strapped to the table. The mask that I have to wear gets strapped to the table and is tight as hell. It's made of a plastic mesh so I'll always have lines on my face after each session. I don't know if I was dreaming, but I swear I smelled burning or something during the session. Maybe they fried something (hopefully the remains of the tumor.) I actually fell asleep during the session. The facial expression on my mask kinda looks like Han Solo in the carbonite… my mouth was a little open when they fitted me for it. I didn't do it on purpose, but with the added pressure to my lips, the mouth automatically opens. This probably explains the physics for French kissing… ha ha ha!

Anyways, I am trying to walk more at home… still have difficulty with the ataxia in my left arm and leg…. I can't wait to get out of this wheelchair… running the race in April might be a long shot but it's something to aim for… The tomotherapy will probably cost me some fatigue and some hair. I am starting to get really bored at home… I'm usually in bed by 10 PM.

Thursday, January 26, 2006

I'm starting to shed hair. My hair is gonna be patchy but I won't lose everything. I think I only lose hair where the radiation enters/exits my head. It doesn't hurt at all. The hair just falls out, no pain at all. It kinda looks like my dog Mercury's fur shedding. Maybe if I was a girl, I'd freak-out a little more. Luckily my hair is really short. The radiation therapy makes me really tired, wipes me out for at least an hour after each session. Today I was able to walk from the car to the waiting room with the walker. I can't wait till this is all over…

Wednesday, February 8, 2006

Whoa… it's been a while since I've updated this thing. I'm hanging in there. This past week has been kinda tough. The radiation is finally starting to take its toll. I caught a little cold last week so I'm gonna lay low for a little while. I'm kinda bummed because I still need that damn wheelchair, but I'm getting around much easier with the walker. I wish I would wake up one morning and everything would be better. Too bad it doesn't work that way. I continue to make improvements, but it's not happening as quickly as I would like. Maybe after radiation is over, things will be more "normal."

I've always dreamed big. But I'm starting to have doubts about that race in April. I literally have to walk before I run. Dude, I can't wait for this to be over. The doctor said 6 months to a year.

Tuesday, February 14, 2006

Radiation is now officially done!!! They gave me a certificate and a hug as well. I kept the mask by the way...I don't know why. They'll make me a new one if I need to come back. I get another MRI in 3 months and follow up with the docs in one month.

Now I can just focus on walking. I just started walking in the parallel bars without a walker or cane. I'm getting rid of the wheelchair going to my remaining appointments on Friday, though I think I'll still keep it around for longer trips.

Also just found out one of my friends from PT school secured tickets for the Pistons-Lakers game at the Staples center. Hopefully I'm on a cane by then. Oh yeah, even though radiation is over, I still don't like Valentine's Day.

This whole experience made me realize that no two people will experience things the same way. I have to follow up with the radiologist every 6 months to monitor what's left of the tumor. Anyways after radiation ended, I was in for the long haul... I thought I had at least one more "stop" before going back to work. This is where my patience and will would really be tested... continued outpatient therapy.

# Ready or Not

Now that I escape, sleepwalker awake
Those who could relate know the world ain't cake

**-The Fugees, *The Score* 1993**

I was discharged from rehab to home in the wheelchair. I still couldn't walk with the walker without minimum assistance. I had outpatient physical therapy and occupational therapy 3 times a week for over 6 months. I also had to do 6 weeks of radiation therapy, which in hindsight probably held me back.

Each week I had a new challenge. Whether it was walking to the elevator or ascending/descending a flight of stairs, it was very important to have weekly goals to monitor my progress for myself. If I came up short of those goals, then I would attack the goal even harder the following week. Common everyday activities were huge missions. Just getting out of bed in the morning to go to the bathroom took forever.

There were a lot of things I wasn't ready for. I was not expecting a simple trip to the bathroom to be so intimidating. After my confidence grew moving around on my own, I started to feel like I should be doing more on my own. The following are excerpts from my personal journal/blog when I first got home. It really helped that I knew my prognosis. It would have helped if I knew someone who had gone through something similar... new, undiscovered territory for me, my family, and my friends.

Sunday, December 11, 2005

My first day home was pretty uneventful. The first thing I did... take a 2 hour nap. Next thing I did was take off that annoying hospital ID wrist band. That thing had been on for weeks!!! I was calling it my prison handcuff because I couldn't take it off and I couldn't leave the building. I missed Thanksgiving. I'm speculating that my insurance probably thought that if I was able to go home, I could just stay home. I was a little bummed I couldn't go home for Thanksgiving.

There are always unexpected obstacles once you get home from the hospital. The biggest thing I was worried about was living with my parents again. I would go from living on my own to potentially getting treated like a child again. Oh well, at least they're here for me. I'm pretty lucky actually, but I'll probably get annoyed so I'll welcome any calls or visitors over the next few weeks…

Tuesday, December 27, 2005

Things are going well. They finally gave me a walker to use at home. I'm standing at the counter for 15 to 30 minutes now. I try to stand as much as I can… I walked a little bit at the mall today with the walker. The biggest things holding me back are coordination, balance, and facial nerve numbness (which affects my speech)… Actually I got discharged from outpatient speech last Monday. Strength and cognition are both good and approaching normal, but coordination is the biggest hurdle. I should be walking with a cane in no time… am actually thinking about signing up for a race (Carlsbad 5000) in April (who's with me???)

Anyways Christmas was cool. The whole family was here. My brother was cracking me up the whole weekend. Way too funny… Definitely a well needed break from my over-protective parents.

Sunday, January 15, 2006

I'm finally getting out more. Last weekend went out on Friday and Saturday with some of my old friends from Michigan, and this weekend I was able to go to a wedding. Thing is, I am still in the wheelchair. I feel like either a second-rate human or a little kid. One or the other. It was weird at the wedding because it was the first time I've seen a lot of my friends since the surgery. I wasn't sure how people would react to the wheelchair.

For the wedding at the church I had to sit in the designated "handicapped area" with the little kids. I didn't mind it though because little kids amuse me. However, it does suck having to look up to everyone to hold a conversation. It also is a pain in the butt asking people to move out of the way if you want to pass by and get to "point b." I know, I know "in due time," "patience." Don't even get me started on the parents… maternal "concern" and rehab don't make a good combination. Anyways, I found out last week I have a hard time taking shots. I'm still gulping my drinks. Beer is not a problem. Last Friday went down to Pacific Beach and met up with some coworkers at a bar for drinks. We ended up at some club. We would have gone to more places, but both places we visited were one level establishments with no steps or stairs. It's OK for me to drink in moderation because I'm not taking any medication and this is what I would normally be doing.

In PT school, I had to do a "wheelchair experiment" (see appendix). Basically I spent a day at the mall in a wheelchair to see what it's like. I found that people in my age demographic ignore me, while the older generations look at me in shame. I got stared at by little kids a lot. They looked scared of me. None of this changed the past 2 weekends when I would go out. What I wasn't prepared for were all the transfers, for example, transferring to different cars, toilets, chairs, and couches.

I hate drawing attention to myself, but it felt like everyone was staring at me whenever I would go out… maybe I'm paranoid or something.

I tried walking into church today (~45 yards and 2 steps with a rail)… yup that's right, I'm a regular there now!!! Still using the wheelchair inside the church if I need it. Not too bad!!! Only a few more weeks and I should be out of that damn wheelchair!!!! Will start week 3 of radiation this coming week.

Going to Catholic Church is very "therapeutic." "Therapeutic" obviously for spiritual reasons, but also it involves a lot of sit to stand transfers and kneeling. I haven't tried kneeling yet, but soon. Anyways, I should be losing my hair from the radiation in the next couple if weeks. I really don't care, but it will be a reminder of how real this thing is. I still have no real side effects from the radiation so far. I have noticed though that I am pretty sleepy when I get out of the Cave. Maybe it's because I usually fall asleep in there and I have a hard time waking up. I've never been a morning person. This is probably the reason I don't normally take naps. Other than that no vomiting, headaches, or pain... not yet...

Sunday, January 22, 2006

Got "Connect-four" from one of my friends from PT school. We used to play every night as a study break. What a great gift! I have yet to lose! Makes me practice reaching with the left hand and helps me strategize. Walked into church today with the walker and left the wheelchair in the car for the first time... took me 10 minutes... only a matter of time now, but I'm starting to get frustrated. I also think I'm starting to get "irritable."

This weekend was pretty laid back. Just got back from watching football at a friend's place. I'm so tired right now... got a busy week coming up. Week 4 of radiation starts this week. My cousins from the Midwest are coming in this weekend. It should be fun!!!

Thursday, January 26, 2006

It's been 3 months since my surgery. Things are going well, but slower than I expected. I just started walking with a single-point cane in the parallel bars. I have a lot of work to do if I want to run that race in April. I'm definitely doing more walking now, but I still need the wheelchair when I go out, because it takes me forever with a walker to go from "point a" to "point b."

I've been having weird dreams as of late. I dream I'm walking around everywhere. I've never wanted anything so badly. When I used to people watch, I used to notice only the hot girls. Now I look at every person's gait pattern with envy. Pretty pathetic. Sigh... in due time...

Friday, February 3, 2006

It sucks knowing what needs to be done, but you're unable to do it. This is the one major drawback of being both a therapist and a patient. It's so frustrating. It's like knowing the winners of the Super Bowl, World Series, and Stanley Cup and not having enough money for a minimum bet.

Initially, I thought I would be ready for a 5K run/walk 5 months after surgery. Today I had my first doubts. I don't think I'm walking enough. It's time to think of some short term goals. Maybe…

1. Going out and walking with the walker without the wheelchair.
2. Walking to the waiting room in therapy sessions with a single point cane.
3. Going to the bathroom with the walker only.
4. Getting a drink out of the fridge.
5. Walk up a flight of stairs with the least restrictive assistive device.

For the first time since the surgery my confidence is being tested.

Monday, February 20, 2006

This weekend I finally went out to dinner without the wheelchair to some Indian buffet. It was so cool seeing my friends again. I was never a huge fan of Indian food but that buffet was awesome! Maybe it was the company… that was the latest (9PM) I've walked in the past 3 months! I wish I could have walked a little faster for everyone there. It felt good getting out of the house for something other than therapy for once.

Anyways, things are going well with the rehab. Walking with the walker is much faster, but I feel like it is slowing me down. The ataxia on the left side is still there but better controlled.

Walking is definitely getting easier. I finally took some steps with the cane outside of the parallel bars from the PT gym to my occupational therapy appointment... wasn't too bad. I can walk with the walker from the front door of the condo to my parking space (>300 feet). I still think I'll be on the cane exclusively in a few weeks. I haven't tried turning around yet... but soon. If I'm off the cane in mid-March things will be looking good for the Carlsbad 5000. Will take a lot of work though.

I have another MRI scheduled on Saturday morning... not as scary or as big deal anymore... I have a feeling I'll be back on the steroids for the swelling. I'm still not on any medications. I keep telling myself this will be over soon. I'm starting to think no one really knows for sure. I can see the light at the end of the tunnel now, but how much further do I have to go?


Saturday, February 25, 2006

Today is my 4-month anniversary of my surgery. This morning I had another MRI of my head. It took about an hour to finish the test. I remember my first MRI and all the anxiety that went along with it. This time I slept through the whole thing. I don't think I'm a tough guy just yet. They called me at 9:00 AM to let me know there was an opening at 9:45 AM. I had to rush out of the house to get there on time. I was still in bed when they called! Usually it takes me an hour to get ready in the morning. I skipped breakfast which is usually either waffles or a bowl of cereal with a protein shake.

Anyways, I took a peek at the MRI films. They look pretty good. There is still a little swelling. I wonder if my neurosurgeon is gonna put me back on the steroids... It's so cool knowing what to look for...

So anyways, today is the 4-month anniversary of my surgery. (Oct. 25, the same day as Lance Armstrong's brain surgery for his tumors.) Anyways, 25 has always been one of my favorite numbers. 25 was my high school football number. Rocket Ishmail wore 25 at Notre Dame while I played HS football. The square root of 25 is a whole number. Multiplication, addition, and subtraction of 25 are easy calculations. That's why I also like the number 9... Easy to calculate the square root and the multiplication rule of 9!

A lot has happened with my friends in the past 4 months. 2 babies were born, one pregnancy announcement, an engagement, a wedding, a new haircut, a new girlfriend, a new car. Man... I've got some catching up to do.

Next weekend I get to see the Pistons in LA... might check out the Red Carpet at the Academy Awards as long as we're there.

Friday, March 17, 2006

I'm finally starting to walk without a cane or walker outside of the parallel bars. The big thing is I need to weight shift forward and laterally when taking a step. I just started standing up in the shower last week. I also just learned how to step into the shower. I'm really starting over. I'm relearning how to walk and how to do basic activities. Simple everyday tasks, like going to the bathroom in the morning, take about 10 minutes. I'm walking with the cane in the hallway with my dad.

I'm such a smartass because I need a reasonable explanation for things whenever someone tells me to do anything, especially my parents. I don't like to listen to my parents because they want me to go slower and safer. My thing is I won't progress if I listen to them. The next goal is to get rid of the walker. Wow, reading my old entries has made me realize how far I've come along and that I've been "out" a really long time. I guess I'm pretty pigheaded and I've been too focused on my goals, which I guess is a good thing.

Wednesday, March 29, 2006

The 5-month anniversary of my surgery has passed. I'm proud to say that things are much better. I've ditched the wheelchair and am starting to walk more with the cane. I'm definitely walking much faster with the walker. I really want to be on that cane soon. Hopefully I'll be walking with nothing by the time my friend's wedding rolls around. I can't believe I'm still the best man.

It seems like any progression I make opens up a whole new world of problems. The thing is, with every step forward I take, I notice how time consuming common everyday tasks have become. For example: clipping my fingernails, showering, eating with a spoon and fork, walking, and putting on pants standing up. There is probably more stuff, but I haven't figured everything out yet.

The Carlsbad 5000 is coming up pretty soon. I still wanna do that race with the cane, but the walker might be the best option... I have this annoying habit of getting really dizzy in PT after working hard for 40-50 minutes. Maybe this weekend I'll try walking a mile at Harbor Island. I still think there is something vestibular going on...

Things were progressing nicely, but not fast enough for me. For the first time I was not able to reach one of my goals. I decided not to do the 5K unless I could walk it. One of my co-workers urged me to do the race in the chair, but I'm a pretty stubborn guy. I promised myself that I'm not gonna do another race until I can at least walk it. My rehab continued much longer than I anticipated, but at least I was using the wheelchair less. At least I was at home now and handled all the unexpected challenges. Oh well, I guess I will do another few months of rehab...

# Don't Stop Believin'

Don't stop believin'
Hold on to the feelin'
Streetlights people

**-Journey**, *Escape* 1981

I was out of that wheelchair and on my feet more frequently. I thought it would only be a matter of time before I could go back to work. I was starting to get frustrated at how long this was taking. Things were finally starting to get to me. People were getting annoying. This was most evident at our family reunion on an Alaskan Cruise. My therapists were telling me that I still had a long way to go before I could return to work. That was hard news to take, but it made me work even harder.

I was less frequently updating my journal/blog because I started to feel like people always knew what was going on with me, but I had no idea what was going on in their lives. I preferred actually talking or emailing people to give them updates on my progress. The journal/blog served its purpose. I worked my butt off trying to research my next goal, walking a Charity 5K. The following are entries to my personal journal and blog as I was waiting to get back to work.

Friday, March 24, 2006

I'm on my feet even more. More walking with/without the cane and walking much faster with the walker. I'm still slower then the old ladies, but I am faster. Jeez, I must have been **really** slow before. It's really humbling getting passed up by little old ladies. I'm noticing the dizziness more frequently if I go from sitting 15 minutes to standing. Like I said I'm more active, so maybe I'm noticing the dizziness more. I'm also noticing things aren't as easy as they used to be.

I spent 45 minutes in OT today trying to put on a pair of pants standing up. I've been getting dressed sitting down this whole time. Tying a towel around my waist after a shower is not as easy as it used to be.

One of the funniest things I had problems with was tying a towel around my waist after a shower. I had just started using the walker more independently. I wanted to walk out of the bathroom with the walker. I did what I normally do: I tie a towel around my waist then I get dressed in my room. The problem was I hadn't practiced this yet in OT. I opened the bathroom door pretty easily, but I hadn't tied the towel tight enough around my waist. As soon as I stepped out of the bathroom, I felt the towel start to loosen and begin to slide down my hips. I mentioned before how much I hate being naked in front of myself. I guess I'm pretty shy. "If I just go a little faster… I can make it to my room." About halfway to the bedroom the towel was completely off! I was now faced with the dilemma do I turn around or continue forward? "Maybe if I'm really quiet and quick no one will notice. Screw it! I'm going to my room."

Soon, I was buck-naked holding nothing but the walker. I was trying to walk as fast as I could, but I was still going at a snail's pace. I think I discovered a new kind of gait pattern, "Naked Walker Walking." Luckily no one saw me. What the hell was I doing? Talk about vulnerable. It makes me laugh now thinking about my "Naked Walker Walking" experience. It seemed like I was buck-naked forever! I'm sure this happens to older people all the time. Eewww! What an ugly mental picture! I quickly figured out that it's much easier if I bring in boxer shorts with me to the bathroom before the shower.

My uncle from Toronto is with me now for the next 2 weeks while my Dad is back in MI taking care of business. My uncle from Florida and my aunt from New York are here for a few days as well to look after me. I always give my guests a week to get used to being around me. I'll let them "baby" me for a little while, but after the week is up I'll start getting sarcastic. I really hate it when people are too helpful.

It makes me feel like I'm completely useless. I'm used to doing things on my own. I hate it when people assume I can't do certain things. It really pisses me off and motivates me even more. If you want to get me fired up, tell me I can't do something and I'll do it just to prove you wrong.

Monday, May 01, 2006

Damn it. I'm still not 100% yet. It's been six months since the surgery and I have nothing but hope pushing me forward. To put it in a sports analogy, I feel like I'm up 3-1 in a best of 7 series. I know I will win in the end, but it's taking longer than I expected and there is a little uneasiness about winning the series. I just wanna get back to work so there is a sense of normalcy again. I've already lost half a year; I don't want to lose anymore time. All I know is I'll be ready for the wedding Memorial weekend. I have to be ready. I'm the best man.

I'm trying to start a new routine. I've gone to Harbor Island a few times to get my endurance up and to practice walking with the cane with the help of my friends. I can go 4 trash cans now (about 100 yards). Without fail, I get words of encouragement from complete strangers. I really appreciate the kind words, but I'm just doing what I need to do to get back on my feet. I feel like I need people standing beside me more than I need them behind me. The words of encouragement are great, but I think I'm getting numb to it. I think things mean a lot more when I get treated like a normal person. Last month a bum told me to "fuck off." It brought a smile to my face.

Old people are my biggest fans. They are always watching and "cheering" for me during my therapy sessions. Which is cool and all, but I'm at the point right now where I ignore it. I've always been taught to respect my elders, so I would never tell them to back off. Actually, some of my best rehab buddies are patients my parents' age. I really feel like I have aged at least 20 years since this whole thing started. Maybe this will help me grow up... nah, I'll still be laughing at monkeys and dick/fart jokes for a while.

**Sunday, June 04, 2006**

Its been over 7 months since the surgery. My will still hasn't been broken. My eyes are still focused on returning to work ASAP. PT and OT are twice a week now. I'm going to be doing a lot more on my own... It's time to start treating myself. I'm gonna start going to the gym at my apartment. I will continue going to church at the Mission San Diego to walk up and down the hill and to walk on uneven ground.

I tried swimming yesterday. It was ugly. No coordination at all. I stayed in the shallow end, but it is a lot easier walking in deeper water. I had my dad with me at the time. He worries too much. He's more scared of me falling than I am. I'll try going to the pool again later this week.

After the wedding I found out I can do shots again. Oh boy...

**Wednesday, June 14, 2006**

I'm really hating the wheelchair now. I feel like I get depressed whenever I'm in it. The way people look at you. I think I just don't like getting pushed around. I feel so helpless. I don't like that at all.

I also hate when people start talking to my dad or anyone with me about me. "Hello, I'm right here." My new "functional goal" in OT should be flipping people off with my left hand... ha ha ha... just kidding!

**Wednesday, June 28, 2006**

I'm on a cruise ship in Alaska right now for a family reunion. My Ninang (Filipino godmother) paid for me. No computer right now. Will have to do this the old-fashioned way, by hand. It's good though; I need to practice writing anyways. To appease my parents I brought the wheelchair with me on this trip. Not sure if I'm having fun yet. I stick out like a sore thumb. People keep staring at me. They're not even discrete about it. Totally pisses me off. I'm getting annoyed. This is what I expected. Even my brother and cousins notice the other people staring.

My parents and my aunts are really being over-protective. My brother and I play a game every dinner to count the number of times we catch my mom looking at me. I think we counted over 10 occurrences in a 5 minute period. Sheesh! I was just eating, nothing even remotely dangerous! What's really annoying was the fact that the wait staff cut my meat for me. Sounds harmless, right? Not when they take the knife out of your hand in the middle of you cutting your own meat. I keep telling myself to settle down and not unload on anyone.

I'm staying in tonight. Hit it big at the craps table yesterday. Tomorrow we dock in Juneau, hopefully we see some whales tomorrow. It's so weird here. The sun doesn't go down til 11:30PM.

Friday June 30, 2006

Ooohhhh I'm pissed off. I was walking with the walker in the dance club on the ship. I was going down a step when some big drunk white guy picked me up like a child to "help me" go down a single step. I kept telling him I didn't need help, but he did it anyways. He put both hands under my armpits, and lifted me up like a child with me still holding the walker. Not only was that embarrassing, but a violation of my personal space. I've never wanted to punch someone in the mouth so bad in my life.

When people try to help me transfer it actually creates more problems than helps. It makes the situation very confusing, too many cooks in the kitchen. It also creates an embarassing, loud scene. I know people are just being helpful, but it causes mass confusion. It would be better if the person you're traveling with helped to perform "crowd control." For example, I very easily could have asked for help from one specific person if presented with the opportunity instead of people "rushing to my aid."

I can't stand it when people talk about me to whoever is pushing the wheelchair. "Hello, I'm right here!" This would happen a lot in the elevators. I hate it when people just assume I don't understand them or I can't do anything. Whenever "annoying" people passed by, my brother would say I should mess with them and make them feel awkward. For instance, I should stare back at the people staring and yell, "WHAT? WHAT UP! YOU WANNA TAKE THIS OUTSIDE!" Ha ha ha! I didn't have the balls to do this because most of the guilty parties were older people and little kids.

Thursday, August 10, 2006

Holy crap! It's been 9 months since the surgery. Who would have thought it would have gone this long. I certainly didn't. As a therapist looking at my impairments and where I was a few months ago, I am just now starting to realize the severity of my surgery. Months have passed and another birthday has passed.. I made it, but I'm still hungry! I really don't feel like celebrating anything until I get back to work. On Sept. 1st I'm going into work to shadow one of my co-workers. Just a couple of hours. I really need to get my feet wet again in the PT world. I've been staying busy by starting a number of side projects.

I just had another MRI this morning. This one came with a little more anxiety. This one is going to be compared to my initial post-op MRI to monitor any changes. Man, I hope there is no growth! If there is, bring it on! I'll take it down.

Walking with the cane is much improved. I'm just now trying to incorporate a two-point gait pattern with the cane. Basically for me that means that the cane and my left leg hit the ground at the same time. The right leg then follows through. Sounds pretty simple, but I'm having the hardest time with balance and weight bearing on one leg. This is really important when walking. When I walk it is really slow. I have to really think about all of the phases of walking with each step. Things are no longer automatic. I'm now walking up for communion at church. It's kind of annoying, though, because my dad is always holding my gait belt whenever I try walking. When we first started he had a tendency to pull on the belt, which would make me lose my balance and cause us to argue about how much help I needed.

Friday, September 01, 2006

I went into work today for the first time with the cane. I was hoping to shadow one of my co-workers, but there were so many "red tape" and liability issues that I forgot about. My dad went in anyways for his scheduled massage, so I sat in the waiting room for an hour. It was a very familiar but weird feeling. I would watch familiar faces pick up their patients and take them back for their treatment sessions. Man, I wished I was in their shoes.

I've sat in waiting rooms for other appointments, but this one was a little stranger because when I worked at the hospital, I would just go to a patient's room. At the outpatient clinic, we go to the waiting room and pick up our patients. Some therapists go all the way in to pick up their patients. Some therapists wait at the entrance of the gym area for their patients to come to them. Here again, is that concept of "control." I really believe that for the first few sessions a therapist should go into the waiting room to establish a strong rapport with their patients. I don't think I've ever sat in our waiting room before. I chose to sit by the door because I felt like I shouldn't be there. It was like sitting in a "restricted area." I kind of felt the same way at the neurosurgeon's office. Actually one time, a lady sitting across from me recognized me as a therapist that worked with her. I remembered her, too; I couldn't do anything for her back pain. I tried not to make eye contact with her. I felt a little embarrassed because I felt like I didn't belong. Sitting in the waiting room for an hour is something every therapist should try at least once. If you get a cancellation and have the time, try it. Put yourself in a patient's shoes. Size up your clinic. The first impression of a therapist or a clinic is built in the waiting room.

Tuesday, September 5, 2006

A few days ago I wasn't sure if I was gonna do the Angel Adventure Charity 5K walk to benefit the National Brain Tumor Foundation (NBTF), but everyone's show of support has given me the confidence to do it! Two of my friends already signed up as members of "Team Galvez." I told them I was only thinking about doing it. I guess I just needed a little push to do this walk. I haven't even walked a mile yet, but I think I can do it.

Friday, September 8, 2006

I've been lying low the last few months. Now it's time to start making things happen! There is a constant battle being waged right now in my head. The tumor is gone (for now), but it pits the young confident athlete in me versus the calm level-headed physical therapist. I keep wanting to do things on my own although I probably still need a little help. The only things holding me back according to the young confident athlete are my balance and coordination. The calm levelheaded PT knows that there are still things that I haven't even tried yet, but progress is still being made. It doesn't help that I'm stubborn and people keep advising me against certain things. I try them anyways. I must have fallen at least 10 times this summer trying stupid things. I'm getting better at correcting my losses of balance. Luckily, I haven't had any major accidents. I'm kinda rooting for the young confident athlete.

A typical day for me starts at 8AM. I still need the walker to walk to the bathroom. Lying down or sitting for longer than 15 minutes gives me a feeling of unsteadiness. I then walk to the kitchen to have my protein shake and waffles. I prepare them myself when I can. I usually eat my breakfast at the counter because it's too much work right now carrying things to the table. After breakfast I go to my room and check my email. I usually have my therapy appointments from 10-12 on Mondays and Wednesdays, so we are out the door at 9:20 so I have time to walk to the garage and time to walk into my appointments. On the days I don't have therapy I have the same morning ritual, but I go to either the Mission San Diego to practice walking on hills, uneven ground, and stairs or walk a lap around my complex. When we get back, I have lunch then jump online again. I usually take a nap around 3, and wake up in time to go to my complex's fitness center to ride the recumbent bike and walk on the treadmill. I'm usually on the machines for 10-15 minutes depending on how tired I am. After that I shower and then have a late dinner. That was my whole summer in a nutshell. Pretty boring, but I know improvements were made! Still not there yet, but I feel like I'm closer to the end of the tunnel. The first major test is that 5K walk.

Friday, September 22, 2006

Dude, I think I'm onto something! Kids are extremely resilient creatures, especially when it comes to achieving "motor milestones" such as walking, running, jumping, or going to the bathroom. I've got the going to the bathroom part down, but the walking thing is giving me fits! Kids show no fear when it comes to doing what they want. That's the kind of fearlessness I need. I figure since everyone treats me like a child anyways, I should look at the human developmental model to progress. Sometimes I think too much when I'm doing a certain activity. I need to stop thinking and start doing! I've been using the treadmill at home (against the advice of a lot of people) to recruit the "central pattern generator" so that I establish a more normal walking pattern. The origins of the "central pattern generator" are rooted in the stepping reaction, which is first present in 1-3 month old infants. We are born with this "stepping reaction." If you hold a baby under his arm pits, and let his feet touch the ground, you'll see the stepping reaction. The legs automatically come up like a regular walking pattern. As we get older, our muscles get stronger and we develop the balance to walk. That is where I am right now. I wanna try running next because I have trouble weight shifting forward when I'm walking. You have to shift your weight forward when running, otherwise you aren't going anywhere. The major problem with running is the fact that for a brief moment both feet are off the ground. Maybe if I try jogging, it will be safer. I wanna try this soon!

Wednesday, October 04, 2006

I'm really getting tired of people telling me I can't do something... I hate to admit it, but I'm starting to believe them. All my therapists don't think I'll be back at work by the end of the year. My dad is constantly questioning my judgement. He always wants me to take the safest route, but at the same time gets frustrated by the slow progress. "Just use the walker," "Turn around and go back," "You can't do that walk," "Just walk later." I feel like I need to push the envelope to progress, try a few things outside of my comfort zone. I hate to say it but if I listened to what people tell me to do, I wouldn't be where I am right now. My confidence is starting to waiver a little, but reality is starting to sink in.

Friday, October 6,2006

I just started hippotherapy today! "Hippos" is Greek for horse, so no, I didn't go to the zoo. Hippotherapy involves using a horse's movements to simulate the normal gait pattern when walking. Basically, you sit on the horse and use your core muscles to keep you on the horse. When the horse walks, since there is no saddle, the hips move the same way as the horse! Just sitting on a moving animal is a lot of abdominal and back work! Again, the movement of the horse simulates the movements of the human pelvis with walking. Things I really need! Hippotherapy has much research in medical journals that document gait improvements in kids with cerebral palsy, so I always thought this it was for kids! Hey, at this point I'll try anything.

Thursday. October 12, 2006

I'm walking a lot further now. Last weekend at Harbor Island I walked about 1K with the cane, and 1K pushing the wheel chair. I'll definitely be ready for the 5K next weekend. Walking for me requires a lot of concentration. A few months ago just getting my left foot to land where I wanted it was a huge task in itself. Here is a list of things I need to consciously remind myself as I'm walking:

1. **Stand up straight - tighten your stomach and extend your back**
2. **Weight shift a little laterally with each step**
3. **Remember the sequence: cane-left foot-right foot**
4. **Keep your back and hips in extension**
5. **Keep your momentum forward, not lateral**
6. **Take a small step with the left leg (only about the length of one shoe)**
7. **Hit the ground with your heel first**
8. **Take a bigger step with the right foot**

There is a lot to think of, so if I get distracted or too tired my walking goes to hell. Most of the time I get distracted when someone sneaks up on me to "cheer" me on. I also get distracted when a cute girl smiles at me. So if I fall, there is usually a cute girl in the area! Ha ha ha!

Saturday, October 14, 2006

I rode the horse again yesterday, except this time I rode "Ginger" backwards. Today I'm noticing my back is a little more sore than the first time I went. Riding backwards really forces me into lumbar extension. I've always been a "sloucher" (bad posture indicated by sitting in a posterior pelvic tilt). You can't slouch sitting backwards on a horse. I really like the dynamic balancing involved with the hippotherapy.

Sunday, October 22, 2006

The charity walk was a huge success! "Team Galvez" raised over $11,000 for the NBTF! We got a cool glass trophy and a few prizes for being the top fundraising team in Orange County. Who would have thought... At first, my competitive juices were flowing and this fundraising thing became a competition for me. I then realized that many of the teams we were "competing" against were teams walking in honor of loved ones lost to brain tumors. Then I figured with the more funds we raise, everybody wins.

Well, the walk itself was fun! 16 people for "Team Galvez" showed up for the walk. I had everyone on the team wear a sports jersey of his/her favorite team. Everyone expected me to wear my Michigan football jersey, but I decided to wear my old JEDI basketball jersey. The JEDI was a basketball team I played on with my friends. Unfortunately, everyone was the same height and we all played similar positions, so we didn't win very many games, but we sure had fun!

Anyways, I finished the walk in 2 hours, enough for a last place finish. I've never finished last in anything. I DON'T LIKE IT! I made up a few rules to make the walk more fun for everyone. *1) Whenever people heard or said: "Eric" or "Galvez," people had to bark like a dog.*

This quickly turned into the Arsinio cheer or if you're too young to remember that, the Randy Jackson Dog Pound, *2) "Tumor" - Hug the closest teammate.* It was funny watching people participate! I just like watching socially awkward situations. Everyone there got to know each other pretty well after the walk, *3) "Walk" - Spank your own butt.* I just wanted to see my dad spank himself! I wanted revenge for years of me being naughty. Of course, I would abuse these rules whenever I could! Hilarious! Ha ha ha!

I crossed the finish line without the cane or wheelchair to a huge ovation from my teammates. We got back just in time for the awards ceremony. I honestly didn't know there were going to be prizes for the top fundraising team. There were so many teams bigger than us! When they called our name I was really surprised! At the end, they called all the brain tumor survivors to the microphone stage. Talk about uncomfortable. First off, I hated being in the wheelchair. Secondly, I have always hated getting my picture taken! I'm more of a "behind-the-scenes" type of guy. Finally, I didn't like being the center of attention for something I consider "just getting back on my feet."

After the walk, the team went to some sports bar to catch the Michigan-Iowa game. Honestly, I think I enjoyed the 2 ice cold beers more than the awards. They totally hit the spot after a long morning. I guess I'm a pretty simple guy. Next year, we'll probably do it again. Hopefully, it doesn't take 2 hours!

After months of planning I was finally able to do something I wanted to do. More importantly, my confidence was back. Well, one more goal to go! I had to figure out a way to get back to work!

# Back in Black

Back in black
I hit the sack
It's been too long
I'm glad to be back
Yes, I'm let loose
From the noose
That's kept me hanging about

**-AC/DC**, *Back in Black* 1980

Ever since I got home from the hospital I just wanted to go back to work. I loved my job! As a physical therapist I got to use science, anatomy, and interpersonal skills everyday to help people achieve their personal rehab goals. Two things that gave me the most pleasure in life were exercising and helping people. Physical therapy would be the perfect profession for me! I could share my knowledge with other people who needed help. I would "team up" with a patient and together we would try to beat each of their physical impairments. No patient was textbook, so each person brought a new challenge. I loved that! I used many of the traditional "guidelines" I learned in school, but each activity/exercise we did was geared towards that unique individual. I got so much personal satisfaction from helping people, plus I would get to know each person I was working with pretty well. I would go home everyday and feel like I actually made a difference in another person's life. Maybe a teacher or a charity worker gets this same kind of personal satisfaction.

I still consider myself a "newbie" because I feel there is so much more I need to learn. Grad school was long and grueling, but the classes were a lot more interesting than the "weeder" classes I took as an undergrad. I actually wanted to go to class because I held an interest in what we were learning. There is only so much you can learn and retain in school. Experience is the best way to learn anything. School will lay down the foundation, but nothing can beat learning from experience. I digress.

So anyways, I was independent getting around with the walker. That was great, but not if I wanted to go back to work. If I worked a desk job things would be fine. I'm confident I would have been back at work sooner, but I can't picture myself sitting behind a desk all day! My standing balance had to be a lot better. The following are my personal journal entries as I prepared myself for the return to work.


Saturday, August 19, 2006

I'm going to shadow one of my co-workers at the outpatient orthopedic clinic for a few hours in a couple of weeks. I'm expecting a few problems at work.

1. **I'll be slow with the cane.**
2. **I have a hard time getting started walking with the cane if I sit too long.**
3. **Speech is a still a little slow. Will people hear/understand me in a busy room?**
4. **Dynamic balance with turning and walking could use some more work.**
5. **Sit - stand transfers on a rolling stool.**

I have 2 weeks to prepare for these problems. If worst comes to worst I'll just use the walker when I go back.


Friday, September 01, 2006

Well, things didn't go quite as I had planned. I ended up sitting in the waiting room while my dad got his scheduled massage at the clinic. I took the cane though. I called my boss yesterday to see if it was OK for me to come in. He told me "no" and asked me if I thought I could go back to work anytime in the near future. That was a shot of reality.

My therapists have been saying this for quite awhile, but maybe I needed to hear it from another source to drive it home. The confident, athletic, young guy in me thinks it will only be another month, but the cool, level-headed physical therapist in me understands it might still be a while. Those two guys are constantly fighting. Anyways, the physical therapist won this round. I forgot about all the "red tape" and liability issues involved if I did shadow someone in the clinic. There's always a chance I could fall, but I feel like I can get around independently with the walker. I'm almost there with the cane, but I have a hard time getting started if I sit for too long. I'll try again in a few weeks. Maybe I can write a waiver so that I don't hold them responsible if something does happen. I'm still rooting for the confident, athletic, young guy.

Wednesday, October 04, 2006

Oh boy, I see clouds on the horizon. My state disability funding just ended. I should be fine financially until December. How am I gonna pay my bills? There is always the chance that this book will sell, but that is not guaranteed. That would be nice, but not realistic. I really don't know if I'll be ready to return to work as a physical therapist by the end of the year. My therapists don't think it's realistic. I can only trust their judgment, even though my confidence is saying I can do it! I've got to start thinking of other avenues. The prospect of case management has come up more then once. Maybe I could go into health education. I have to be realistic but still keep my eyes on the prize. I will eventually be a PT again, but I have to do something in the meantime to pay the bills.

Friday, October 13, 2006

I figured out a way to stay here. I called my Long-term Disability plan (private insurance from my health plan), and it should be enough to cover my expenses out here! I also applied for social security disability, but that is a long process. The LTD should get me through another year although I want to return to work before the end of the year. At least I don't have to move back with my parents. I can just focus on returning to work. I am looking more into case management or maybe insurance utilization.

Wednesday, October 25, 2006

Wow, a year ago I had massive brain surgery. Last year, my biggest concerns were the Foley catheter and making it out of surgery. Now the biggest thing on my mind is getting back to work!

Thursday, October 26, 2006

I've been trying to talk to people to brainstorm an interim job before I return to physical therapy. Case management has come up a few times, but I am feeling a lot of hesitancy from some people. Nobody has told me outright that it's not a good idea yet, but I know that's what they are thinking. With case management a lot of walking is involved, talking on the phone, and organizing discharge meetings. To address those potential problems… I think that if I use the walker, I can get around independently. I should be even faster within the next few months. Talking clearly will take some hard work and practice, but I'll work on it. I'm a Type-A personality anyways so I think I can handle the organization. Now, I won't be too familiar with all the nursing aspects of discharge, but I'm willing to learn. Most case managers I know are nurses with solid medical backgrounds and years of experience. I would be pretty young compared to other case managers and I would have limited medical experience, but I think my firsthand experience in outpatient and inpatient therapy would make me a good candidate to be a case manager in an orthopedics or rehab floor. Of course, I can't compete with years of nursing experience, but I'd be willing to learn. All I know is that I don't want to let my medical background and schooling to go to waste. I'd like to work with patients if possible. I can't picture myself sitting at a desk in the same place all day.

Sunday, October 29, 2006

I realize that I need to have a solid back up in case I can't return to work as a physical therapist. I also know that it takes around 2 years for people with spinal cord injuries to accept their disability. A year has passed since my surgery, but I still intend on a full recovery. Jeez, I hope I'm not fooling myself. No one knows the solution to this dilemma. This is a very unique situation according to my doctors and therapists. I'm still making progress, but I'm deathly afraid of hitting a progress plateau. As long as I keep seeing improvement I should be fine emotionally. I think that I should be focusing on short-term goals to monitor my progress. I still can't help but look at a few of my long term goals: I want to start interviewing for new jobs in Dec. This spring I want to run a 5K. This summer I wanna try surfing again.

Monday, October 30, 2006

This weekend my dad went up to San Francisco to visit a friend of his from school, leaving me at home alone for the first time in months. I was glad he was able to go up there because I would be by myself all day on Friday and totally independent over the weekend. I've been waiting for that for months! Although I was by myself I got numerous calls from both my parents. I just let the phone ring, then I would call them back at my own convenience. The only thing I had trouble with was making spaghetti noodles and pouring hot water into the strainer. I didn't burn myself, but it did require a little extra care and thought because I hadn't tried it before. Saturday and Sunday were football days. Overall, I think it went well. No accidents. I can't wait till my next alone time.

Tuesday, October 31, 2006

I'm starting to explore the other work options. I've got a couple leads, but I'm just waiting to hear back from them. I hope I can find something that suits me. I feel like I can still be productive. I really don't want to let my education go to waste. I still intend on going back to work as a PT but it might be awhile. Right now I feel like I need to come up with something to ease my mind.

A year has passed since surgery. Well, I have been diligently working on getting this book published. Hopefully it gets picked up and is the solution to my work dilemma. I'm tired of sitting in the background. I gotta be practical and come up with "plan B." I could just sit back and live off my long term disability for the next year, but I think I would get bored. I am even more focused now on getting back to work as a PT. At least I know now that I can do a lot on my own. The next few months I plan on making things happen! The following chapters are what happen next. The journey was only beginning...

# The Best of You

My head is giving me life or death
But I can't choose
I swear I'll never give in
I refuse

**-Foo Fighters**, *In Your Honor* 2005

This chapter is the beginning of the second year of my journey. I had no idea it would last this long. Time really seemed to have flown by because my eyes were always focused on how I was going to attain the next goal. In fact, I surprised and shocked a lot of people when I published this book and then walked 3.1 miles in a popular 5K race. I figured, "What do I have to lose?" It all just proves that if you want something bad enough you'll get it.

Friday, December 22, 2006

I'm back home in Michigan right now for the holidays. I'm kinda glad to be home because it has been a hectic year. I wasn't able to come home last year, so this year has special meaning. I feel like I come back a wiser man. I'm eagerly awaiting the release of my book. I think it really has good potential because there has never been anything written like it before. At least I haven't come across anything like it. Part of me still can't believe I will actually pull this off. But then again, I really believe if you want something bad enough, you'll get it.

I'm here for 3 weeks. I'm a little ticked off at this because there is a lot of work I still need to do in San Diego. How am I going to practice walking? How will I stay busy here? This is a critical time with regards to completing the book. It's gonna be cold! I think I've lost my Midwestern cold tolerance. I have been spoiled by the warm San Diego sun! This is the last time I will let my mom take care of my travel arrangements!

I've gone to the movies a few times. Walking with the cane in a crowded mall is pretty challenging. I get the same looks from people now as when I was in the wheelchair. But I really don't care anymore. I'll do whatever it takes to get back on my feet. Maybe, the looks come from the fact that my dad refuses to let go of the safety gait belt when I'm walking. I'm still not 100% independent with the cane yet so I understand his concern. He won't let me fall. I think I need to prove to him I won't break.

I went back to my old stomping grounds in Flint with my old roommate from PT school. We stopped by school and I donated my MRI. It was kind of weird to see students sitting in the hallway cramming for practical exams. I remember all the anxiety and shaky hands waiting for those tests. Me and my friend spent 3-4 hours just hanging out in the faculty break room with our old professors.

On Saturday, I hung out with my friends from PT school. Most are married/engaged now and buying houses. I'm still not ready to settle down yet. I think I'm just a late bloomer.

Sunday, December 24, 2006

Saw *Rocky Balboa* on Friday night. Actually, I was pleasantly surprised it didn't suck. My brother, my cousin and I used to follow the Rocky Saga religiously. We knew all the lines from *Rocky III* and *Rocky IV* verbatim. According to my cousin, *Rocky V* never existed. Maybe it's just me but I like watching and reading about underdogs. I could go on about this, but I won't.

Last night I hung out with more friends from PT school. We went to Chelly's Chili Bar and then to some martini bar. I'm not a big fan of martinis so I went with a nice safe frosty Guinness. The bar was kind of crowded, so walking in an unfamiliar place with a nice buzz was a challenge. It sucks having to depend on people for transportation. I felt like a burden on my friends. I wanted to try walking with the cane, but I know I am not ready yet. At least now I know my "theoretical" limitations are real. But since I'm stubborn, I need to experience them first hand.

I think I'm starting to get worried about staying in this condition. I wish someone could give me the answer to this dilemma. It's like all I can do is wait it out.

Monday, January 01, 2007

I'm so glad 2006 is over. I'm ready for a new start in 2007. I've been working on a "secret" project the past year. Check out this site. www.ericgalvezdpt.com. You might recognize a few familiar faces that helped me with this project. It's basically a book based on my blogs from the past year. It's different from anything out there right now because it contains:

1. **The patient perspective from a young active male with a physical therapy backgroud.**
2. **The perspectives of the closest people to me during this life-changing ordeal.**
3. **Information about a "book soundtrack" on iTunes once the book is available.**

I'm excited to announce that the book should be available by the end of the month. Check the website for updates. I've got some cool things planned for 2007. Look out for more updates on the webpage!

Thursday, January 04, 2007

I've been home for almost 3 weeks now. Whenever I come home, I always get really nostalgic. I end up going through old photo albums/ yearbooks and old knick knacks from my room. You take one look at my old room and that's me. *Star Wars* posters, Michigan and Detroit pistons paraphernalia, super hero books, and other junk from high school. It's always kinda cool looking at all those things and realizing how priorities have changed. It's nice seeing my "evolution" through the years. In high school it was all about excelling in sports and getting into Michigan. In college it was learning about myself and testing my limitations. Post college it was getting into grad school. And after grad school it was finding a good job in a place I wanted to be. Last year it was getting back on my feet (literally... ha ha ha!). This year? I'm going to find a way to feel useful again! I have a lot planned for 2007. I think I'm gonna start posting more frequently on www.ericgalvezdpt.com. Who knows where my new project is going to take me?

Thursday, January 11, 2007

Things are starting to get busy. I've been contacted by the Sharp healthcare public relations staff. I'm not exactly sure what they want yet. I've already got some positive comments about my project. Now it looks like things are going to get a little crazy soon. I have also come up with a great marketing idea to promote brain tumor awareness. STICKERS! I figure everyone had a sticker collection growing up. These stickers could be put on iPods, cell phones, laptops, or backpacks. I'll call it "coffee shop or library marketing." Theoretically it sounds like a good idea but we'll see if I can pull this off. The book should be out by the end of the month. I've got some pretty ambitious plans once the book is available. Since I've been home my brother called me out on "neglecting" my rehab. I'm spending too much time concentrating on extracurricular activities, and not enough time working on getting better. He's partially right. That is what led to my lower GPA in undergrad! I'm still having problems with my slower speech and putting my weight on the left leg when standing or walking. I'm trying to do my vocal warm ups from my college a cappela group to strengthen my voice. I'm visualizing "crushing things" with my left foot when I walk to promote putting weight on my left leg.

Wednesday, January 17, 2007

Right now I'm focusing on some new stuff. I'm not looking back until I finish the race. The book is not perfect and I have edited it myself. It is much harder than I thought. I guess you can call it more of a "pure" manuscript complete with mistakes. The next edition should be better once I start it!

(1/20) I'm not a writer. I published this "blook" (book based on a blog) because I felt like it needed to be written. I had a hard time finding resources for young adults in similar situations. The blook is for healthcare students, patients, and their loved ones who had to hear those scary words, "We found a mass in your_____ (insert important body organ here)." Hopefully this spawns more awareness for brain tumor research and inspires someone to write a better book. If you're reading this message, you're probably computer savvy. So, please email all your friends about this site or mention it in your blog/myspace/facebook because well… quite frankly, TUMORS SUCK!

Thanks, Eric


Thursday, January 25, 2007

Thanks to everyone for visiting my site and supporting my crazy project. I have met so many cool people from this. Dude, I really hope you like my "blook." Right now I consider it a manuscript more than a book because I couldn't afford to get it professionally edited. But if it gets picked up by a larger publisher then I'll consider it a real book.

Actually, I've been getting a lot of surprising compliments on my writing style. I didn't even know that I had a style. I'm not a writer. I'm a blogger. (Blame my friend Jon for that.) Seriously, ask me to describe a beautiful tree on a sunny, warm autumn day and my honest response would be one of the following:

1. **It's cool**
2. **It's very cool**
3. **It's nice**
4. **It's very nice**
5. **It's a tree**

Thanks for stopping by. Join me in my fight against brain tumors. Tell a friend about this site. Keep Fighting! Eric

Wednesday, January 31, 2007

Last week I ran some errands with my dad. We were looking at heat exchange pumps for my furnace. Our missions were to find out as much as we could and to find the most reasonable price. On our way to the heating/cooling aisle my dad saw some night-lights he wanted to buy for the kitchen. Since I was using the walker in the store I waived him ahead so he didn't have to wait for me. By the time I got to the aisle he was finishing up his conversation with the sales rep so I turned around and headed back. I waived him ahead again and met him outside.

I found him outside the store having an intense conversation with one of the employees. I noticed he was still holding the nightlights. I couldn't take my eyes off it. He was using it to point at things and "air draw" the size of our broken heat pump. I must have been smiling the whole time because he had no idea that he was still holding them. After his conversation was over and we were walking back to the car, I asked him, "Did you pay for that?" He looked down at his hand, smiled and raced back into the store, leaving me in the parking lot outside of a locked car.

When my dad got back to the car I told him, "We could have just left. It was only a $3 set of nightlights." He insisted going back was the "right" thing to do. How could I argue against that? I've been really lucky to have such good mentors. My dad, Jose Galvez, my mom, Teresita Galvez, my high school teachers, my professors from PT school, and my coaches have all played huge roles in my life. I only hope that someday I can be a positive influence to another human being the same way they were to me.


Sunday, February 4, 2007

I have 2 songs in my head: "*Give Me Novacaine*" by Green Day and "*Breath Through*" by Annie Stela. Preview them on iTunes.

Physical and occupational therapy have officially ended. I really want to run and go surfing this summer. My friends have graciously volunteered to help me after work. My new goals are these:

1. **Run a race this year**
2. **Paddle out to the line up this summer on my surfboard**
3. **Get picked up by a large publisher**

I want to run because I feel like I need some form of competition in my life. Running will only benefit my independence with walking. I figure that if I can do that, then I can handle anything. I really didn't start participating in races until I moved out to San Diego. That feeling of accomplishment, runners' high, is what I miss.

I seriously can't wait to start surfing again either. I wasn't a great surfer before the surgery, but for me it isn't about the act of surfing. Honestly, I used to just enjoy paddling out and sitting on my board waiting for a good wave. It was so chill sitting on my board watching the ocean horizon and shooting the breeze with friends. It was always a struggle getting to the "outside" past the "white wash" waves close to the shore. The reward of sitting on your board with Mother Nature, free of all worries, was well worth the energy expended. That sounds so hippy, but there is no other feeling in the world like it. When I caught my first wave I was hooked.

And the last goal I have is to increase awareness for brain tumor research and the physical therapy profession to the general public. Even though I'm at the tail end of my young adulthood, I also think that young adults are a patient population that often times gets overlooked in favor of the cute "little kids," "established" adults, or the cute "grandparents." It is time the plight of young adult survivors is noticed.


Tuesday, February 6, 2007

Two days ago I received a phone call from someone I haven't seen in a long time. We agreed to have dinner tonight. I just found out the person I was talking to wasn't who I thought it was. The whole time I was talking to someone who I thought was actually someone else. hee hee... Tells you how "deep" my telephone conversations are.

"Sup. Wanna eat? Where? Bye."

So it was my cousin from Canada who called to let me know he was in town for business. He's never called me before. I swear it sounded like a friend of mine. For two days I thought my friend was here and we were gonna have dinner tonight. Two Days! Luckily some friends said something to me and I realized my mistake early! That would have been a really embarrassing situation. I should have been tipped off because I didn't recognize the phone number or the area code. Oh well. It's all good. We're still gonna eat.

Sunday, February 25, 2007

Some crazy opportunities are popping up. I have a friend who wants to write a screenplay based on the book. I have also been nominated to be a graduation commencement speaker at U of M Flint. That has got to be the wildest thing so far! I'm even planning on setting up some book events outside of San Diego.

As for the rehab, things are going pretty well. Some of my friends have agreed to help me after work. I'm walking much better without the cane. I think I still need a hand on me for balance when I walk. I'm also going to the pool every Friday to work on swimming/surfing. The pool is constantly around 90 degrees and is used for therapy classes. I think I am going to be a stronger swimmer than I was before. I'm sitting on the emergency board like a surf board and using a body board to practice kicking. I know I'll be ready for the summer. I started running in the pool on Friday from one end to the other. Running in water is easier than running on land because you un-weight the body in water. Why didn't I think of this before!

I'm going to a year off my career as a PT to promote this book thing. I think it has really good potential, but it makes me nervous knowing its potential. I'm at my computer more than ever before. It's still a little funny because when I'm at my computer I have to have music playing in the background. I'm not a very talkative guy, so my voice is not as strong as it should be. But, I figured out a way to work on that, as well. I just sing along with songs. For some reason the only songs I catch myself singing are The *Backstreet Boys* and *N'Sync*. I only practice this when I'm certain no one will catch me. Dude, I know all the lyrics and "fills" to these songs. I recorded myself on my old tape recorder once. Hilarious!

Sunday, March 4, 2007

Ever since my surprising diagnosis I've been forced to go to church with my family. I consider myself more spiritual than religious. I went to a Catholic grade school, a Catholic middle school, and a Catholic high school. Religion has been forced on me ever since I can remember. I even remember my Lola (grandmother) teaching me the "Our Father" prayer when I first started to speak. But something weird happened over the past year. I finally started really listening in church. Now, I don't mind going to church; in fact, I can't even imagine not going anymore! The "**Mystery of Faith**" is really poignant for me.

- **Christ has died.**
- **Christ is *Risen*.**
- **Christ will *Come Again*.**

As a guy trying to make a "comeback", that is exactly what I wanted and needed to hear. Then I got to thinking about the word "mystery." You don't really know if this is true. Faith in general really is a mystery. For me, it's hard to believe in something that doesn't have solid statistics or facts to prove it. That's why "faith" is a "mystery." You can choose to believe what you want, but I feel F*aith in Something* is essential for a "comeback." For me, I needed this outlet. Religion is a very touchy subject because it deals with an individual's personal beliefs. Just had to get this off my chest.

Wednesday, March 7, 2007

Tomorrow I'll be on TV for the first time. I'll be part of a segment highlighting the different rehab programs at Grossmont hospital. I'll get about a minute of camera time, which is totally fine by me!

Anyways, had my follow up MRI yesterday and I stopped by my old work to pick up a few books. Here is my hypothesis on how things have progressed with me.

1. **The meningioma was a slow-growing tumor. I didn't start experiencing symptoms till I started swimming.**
2. **All the head turning for breathing caused the tumor to bounce around in my head, creating trauma with resulting edema or swelling.**
3. **The edema was well-controlled with the medications: prednizone and dexamethsone.**
4. **Swimming brought things up much sooner. The tumor could have gotten much bigger and the symptoms could have gotten a lot worse years from now. Better now than later, when I have more responsibilities.**

### *Surgery was necessary.*

Now I am dealing with some sort of CNS wallerian degeneration around the nerves associated with the cerebellum, which is why my coordination/balance are messed up. Since the tumor was so close to the cerebellum, something must have gotten damaged. I haven't come across much literature providing positive results about the full regeneration of these nerves. All I am thinking is that there is a first time for anything because I'm still making progress. I'm not giving up! Just a hypothesis, but I'll try to confirm this with the neurosurgeon at my next appointment.

Thursday, March 15, 2007

I'm working on paddling my surfboard in the pool. Also simulating sitting balance on the board, falling off the board, and running in the water. Can't wait to try standing up on it. Standing balance on it is a whole 'nother game. Realistically, I think paddling to the lineup is a more realistic goal.

My brother is coming tomorrow for 2 weeks. He is one of the few people who knows how to push my buttons. My competitive juices flow whenever he's around. I really hope I don't try something stupid and hurt myself while he's here.

The Carlsbad 5000 walk is in 2 weeks. I'm being selfish. No fundraising. This one is just for me.

Tuesday, March 27, 2007

The Carlsbad 5000 is this Sunday. I'm going to be ready. I think I'll walk early in the AM with the Masters runners 40 and older. I'll finish in last place again, but right now I'm more concerned with finishing in two hours. I chose to walk earlier because it won't be as crowded. Plus if I take longer than one hour there is a little more leeway, so I don't have to worry about time. I'm positive I can finish it, but I'm not sure how long it will take. For the record I can go about 1.5 miles in 1 hour, without the cane. I'll probably end up starting with the cane though. We'll see how far I go with it.

As for the crazy stuff I've done so far… I took my first steps without anyone holding, I tried driving electric scooters in Target and Costco. (Was kinda fun, but they don't go very fast), I crossed a busy street for the first time. There will be more stuff on the way. I'm even noticing I'm staying up later and waking up later thanks to Oliver. Still haven't done anything really crazy yet, but there is still a week to go. All it takes from him is "Why not, are you a wuss now?" (That's the "edited Rated G" version.)

Sunday, April 1, 2007

Well, I did it. It took longer then I thought, but it's over now. The Carlsbad 5000 is one of the premier 5Ks in the world (thousands of people run it every year, and they hold 9 separate category races for the large crowds it attracts.) 19 world records have been set there, so it draws the world's elite runners. 2 years ago I set my personal record and earned my first long distance medal for finishing in the top 250 for my age group. Not too shabby for a non-distance runner! I wasn't going to set any personal bests today. I just wanted to finish.

I ended up walking early with the women's masters 40 + at 8AM. I was a little crazy to think I could finish in two hours. It took me three hours to walk the 3.1 miles! The last ½ mile I needed 2 people helping me out. It was nice having my PT friends (Rosalia and Dan) there because I don't know how long it would have taken to finish without them. I really needed to concentrate when walking, but dude…there were so many distractions: People yelling words of encouragement; people staring at me; advice from my both my PT friends; "people watching"… Hee hee! Everyone was really cool with their words of encouragement, for which I am grateful. I was "hamming it up" at the end! Any "GO BLUE" shout I heard was returned with a thumbs up from me! At the finish line I instinctively threw up a "We're #1" finger in the air. In hindsight it was kinda stupid because that gesture should be reserved for championships. I also had a news cameraman and a reporter from the local paper waiting for me. It felt so good getting to the finish line mainly because I was tired as hell, but also because I had tons of people cheering for me! Someone even gave me her medal just for finishing. I really appreciated that small gesture. That medal symbolized so much hard work and commitment from the last year and a half! But I'm still not satisfied because there is plenty of room for improvement and things I need to do

Surfing and running are the next challenges. I want to be at the beach this summer!

Well I returned to the Carlsbad with a little more attention from the spectators and even made the local news. I had a lot planned in the fall so the summer was my selfish time to hit the beach. I figured I should enjoy myself because I figured I would be really busy in the fall. I needed to get back to the beach. The next mission was catching a wave. Not an easy task to do, especially since I was a novice surfer before surgery. The summer brought many new challenges.

# Rollin'

Breathe in now breathe out
Hands up now hands down
Back up back up
Tell me what you're gonna do now
Keep rollin' rollin' rollin' rollin'

**-Limp Bizkit**, *Chocolate Starfish and the Hot Dog Flavored Water* 2000

I started to go out more frequently and was starting to feel more like myself. I started to do more things on my own. I felt more comfortable going out. I also started public speaking, something of which I have always been deathly afraid. I have never liked being alone in the spotlight. My main goal though was to return to the beach to go surfing. I missed the beach. I knew that the fall would be very busy, so the summer was my selfish time. My stubbornness was in rare form this summer.

Friday, April 20, 2007

Yesterday went out with just the cane for the first time. No falls, but I definitely need someone with me when I do that… especially if there is beer involved. I walk like a drunk before my lips even touch an ounce of alcohol. Met up with a bunch of people… actually my OT from the ICU was there. I had so many questions for her because for the 8 days I was in there, I remembered very little. All I remember was opening my eyes a few times and being around different people each time. Thank God I didn't do anything crazy! It was strange hearing stories about myself that I couldn't remember. Apparently, I was really concerned with my butt showing! hahaha! I don't doubt the credibility of that at all.

Saturday, May 12, 2007

Well my first official book event went pretty well. There was a turnout of about 20 people for the lecture, which was what I was expecting due to a beautiful spring weekend in La Jolla. Unfortunately, the books didn't arrive on time, so I just gave the lecture, which lasted about half an hour.

The lecture itself was going to be exciting because as most people know, I'm a quiet guy and I haven't spoken longer than 5 minutes since the surgery! To make matters even more complicated we were having presentation issues from the start. My laptop couldn't connect with the projector and there were issues showing the video I wanted. Luckily most of these problems surfaced yesterday during my run through.

Something strange happened during the presentation. Something that hasn't happened in a really long time. When I started talking about the beginning of my journey, I could start to feel my eyes well up and my voice quiver. I didn't lose it, but it was the first time in a long time that a tear came out of my eye. STUPID ALLERGIES! Just kidding! I was just glad to finally let it out. I just realized it's the first time I've spoken about my journey. I've read my own words many times, but I've never spoken about it! Verbalizing my story kind of brought everything back to the surface. That was long overdue. 18 months of pent up fear, anxiety, and frustration were in those salty little drops of water. Hopefully it doesn't "open the floodgates" like Chandler Bing!

Since there were no books at the event, they invited me back for another event. Hopefully when I give the next lecture I won't have leaky eyes and there will actually be books there. I guarantee the next one will go smoother!

Saturday, May 19, 2007

She's fat and spoiled now. But she's still my girl! She's 8 now, but she'll always be that puppy to me. This is from my blog 3 years ago.

**An Ode to Mercury** (Dr. Seuss-style)

*I took you home in a Xerox box*
*You were so small you fit in my socks.*
*Named you for Mercury Hayes #9*
*The most underrated receiver of all time*

*Wanted to train you to beat up Kal-el,*
*Chris Lum's evil pussycat from hell.*
*He was mean, moody, and he would bite*
*Actually… there's no way you'd win that fight.*

*It's OK because you're still tough*
*Much like yo' daddy but not as rough.*
*I taught you: "sit," "down," and "roll."*
*With my table scraps I filled your bowl*

*For the first two weeks we'd sleep on the floor*
*Then finally I decided, nuh-uh… no more.*
*I used to sleep, on the floor with you,*
*But then I'd wake up next to your poo.*

*Had to let you try it on your own*
*Even tried rewarding you with a bone.*
*Somehow you did it, you fell asleep…*
*Now just stop biting me with your puppy teeth*

*Unfortunately couldn't keep you at townhouse.*
*Somehow the rental management found out.*
*Then I took you home to meet the parents*
*Ma loved you right away, but Papa didn't!*

*You see he's always been scared of little dogs.*
*One bit him hard… in the butt-tocks.*
*It was so funny watching him run.*
*You jumped and you barked, so much fun!*

*Didn't take them long to fall in love with you.*
*Or very long to get dog #2.*
*Rocky, the beagle, that little stinking rat.*
*Does absolutely nothing, he's functionally a cat.*

*I tried to teach you to play fetch,*
*But you wouldn't drop the stick, you little Beee...*
*Hind my back I would hide the stick*
*But you always caught on to my little trick.*

*Then I moved... cross country again.*
*I think Oliver and Rocky are now your best friends.*
*Regret I was never able, to teach you more tricks*
*But you ARE better now at dropping the sticks.*

*I miss the way you greet me at the door.*
*You jump and you bark, you put me on the floor.*
*Sloppy wet kisses all over my face.*
*Tail moving rapidly all over the place.*

*Your mouth always open, as if you are smiling*
*Another fond memory, for me to be filing.*
*I can't wait to see you again in June*
*We'll play outside till we see the moon.*

*Happy Birthday Merc-dawg, I can't believe, you're five years old*
*You're the best-est dog in the whole wide world.*
*Even though you're huge now, I consider myself lucky.*
*A full grown man, coming home to his puppy.*


Sunday, May 27, 2007

Only one more week till I'm out there again! Scoped out the beach already this morning. I'm hoping for 1-3 foot waves and water temperatures around 65. In a perfect world it will be sunny and 75...

but it won't be. Watching other people catch waves has made me even hungier to return to my new hobby. I will have trouble:

- **walking on the sand**
- **bracing myself for the incoming waves**
- **paddling out of the "white wash"**
- **transporting a surfboard to the water**
- **standing up**
- **distractions - people will be watching (I don't like being the center of attention)**
- **putting on the wetsuit**

I'm getting excited! It's going to be ugly, but you have to start somewhere. I already know I'm going to fall, but I will get up every time! If this goes well… guess what I'll be doing this summer to pass the time?

Monday, May 28, 2007

This is also from my blog 3 years ago. Keep in mind I was not a good swimmer at that time. I'm still not.

One word… **amazing**. I've heard people talk about it. **The Rush**. A brief moment of complete calm. You think you see it. You can hear it coming. You start to paddle away. The sound gets louder and louder. You can feel it tilting the board forward under your stomach. The sound is now under you. Is this it? Is it time now? Instinctively you pop up. You're on your feet. You open your eyes. You're standing up. Another brief moment… of terror cause you don't want to fall. You can see the water form odd geometrical shapes around your feet beneath you. Thoughts of sharks and drowning quickly go away. Is this really happening? You look around and it hits you. You're riding your first wave! I still can't believe I popped up on my very first wave. Incredible. Riding something that you have no control over… whoa, I can't even describe it… "Taming" what mother nature throws at you gives you such a rush… **THE Rush**. Dude, I didn't stand up for that long, but it was just a brief taste of what I was looking for, what I've heard so much about... **The Rush**.

Now don't get me wrong, I'm not a surfer yet. After screwing around in the white wash, I tried paddling out farther to catch the outside waves, but I fell off the board into the deep water. Sheer terror. I panicked. My feet couldn't touch the ground, I felt my chest tighten. All my limbs went ballistically out of control. Then I remembered the leash. I reached for the leash around my ankle and pulled the board towards me. Touchdown! As I grabbed for the board... another wave hit... Sheer terror again... Only this time when I grab the board I won't let go. Got to the board... and on my stomach, rode the waves back to the shore. I was done for the day. A harsh slap of reality in my quest for **The Rush**.

Surfing... my new challenge for the summer. Must conquer my fear of the water. I will make the ocean my b*tch. The Classic Conflicts: Man vs Nature. Man vs Self.


Monday, June 4, 2007

Well I made it out yesterday. Even caught a few waves on my knees. I'm too slow popping up to my feet, but I'm sure a little wax will help next time. It felt good catching the waves (even though they were in the white wash.) It was the first time in a long time I had a lot of fun just screwing around. Some of my friends (the "diehards") were there to help me out. I got there early and just wanted to sit in the waves. I crawled on my hands and knees to the water. I didn't care that other people were watching wondering what I was doing. I'd forgotten what the ocean tastes like. I was quickly reminded that I don't like water in my nose. While I waited for my friends, I started out sitting in the water. Soon I was kneeing in the water trying to stay upright fighting the waves. After a while I tried popping up on the sand. This was a huge challenge because

1. **The waves throw off your balance**
2. **Your feet are always sinking in the sand affecting balance again**

I wasn't ready for the speed of the waves. I tried standing up, but I don't think I got up fast enough. Popping up and standing on the floor is really easy, but popping up and standing/balancing on a narrow moving board is a whole 'nother game. Can't wait to try it again!

Wednesday, June 13 2007

Traveled by myself for the first time since surgery last weekend. I can do it, but I need help from the wheelchair pushers at the airport. Everyone is surprised I did it, but come on… would you expect anything less from me? It wasn't so bad. Preboarding before everyone, bypassing long security lines for a pat down, not having to walk in the airport… I figured if grandparents can do it, so can I!

I flew up to northern California to visit my godson and my friends in Mountain House, CA. I got a taste of family life. I'm totally not ready for that, but someday I will be! I haven't been around that many kids since I was one myself. Culture Shock… but very cool! I think THAT is what I want eventually, but right now there is too much on my plate! My godson just turned two, so I got him the Dancing Spiderman. It was so cool watching him dance to it and hearing him laugh. I can't wait until I understand what he is saying!

I think I'm getting some of my confidence back, but at the same time I'm becoming more aware of my limitations. I'm still improving, but knowing what I know about rehab timelines is starting to make me nervous. Actually there are no case studies out there addressing what I am going through, so in a way I feel like I'm breaking new ground. I'm making some good connections through the book. I'm meeting a lot of executive directors and organization leaders. Who knows where those connections will lead me. Some potentially "big" stuff could come out of those connections, but we'll wait and see. My "spidersense" tells me some pretty crazy stuff will happen in the fall. Stay tuned!

Monday, June 18, 2007

Don't laugh too hard. I've been doing a lot of reading lately. Actually I just rediscovered the public library and got my first San Diego library card! I haven't checked anything out of the public library since I was in high school! You know you can "rent" DVDs and other stuff from there for free! That's not the funny part.

So I'm doing a lot more reading now than I ever have. I started reading some of my old books from grad school. I was really fascinated by one book in particular ... *Complementary Therapies in Rehabilitation.* I can't even remember what class it was for, but I think I opened the book once, maybe twice. Most of the topics it touches upon are eastern medicine based... the mind-body relationship. Stuff that is not the focus of traditional western philosophy.

So anyways I decided to give yoga a try... to work on my balance and flexibility. One of my friends agreed to show me a few poses. I told her right off the bat I REFUSE to wear tights. Here's the kicker. Every time I assume a state of relaxation, my mind wanders towards Star Wars and using "the Force." I try to be serious and focus on what I'm doing, but I can't help but crack a smile. Honestly though, my breathing has gotten better and the weight bearing on my left leg has really improved. I think I am more "aware" of my left leg. Hmmmm... the mind-body relationship was never really taught in school. This will require more investigation. **The "Force" is strong in me**. hahaha! Yup, you can make fun of me now!


Monday, June 25, 2007

This week I get to spend all by myself. Both my parents are in Vegas for a reunion. My parents made a very strong push for me to go with them. I refused to go because I would have gotten "babied" there and more pissed off. Hanging out with multiple over-protective Filipino moms is not my idea of fun. I've been waiting for this for about a year and a half. I appreciate everyone's helpfulness, but I'm glad to finally get some alone time. Everyone around me gets to take a break but me.

I'm treating this like a vacation. It's not as easy as I thought. I wanted to make some eggs for breakfast yesterday, but I've got a new "intension tremor" in my right hand. That coupled with the pre-existing ataxia in my left arm makes cooking a little more difficult due to the shakiness in my hands... especially cracking an egg open and hoping not to make a mess. I haven't even tried getting the mail yet, which will require about a 500 foot walk to the mail box. I'm seeing a new neurologist at UCSD next month... he is a movement specialist. I hope he can shine some light on what's going on. I'm still going to do what I want, but dude this is taking forever! I'm really getting tired of "oh you're young, you'll be fine"... Well my cognition is fine, but physically I'm not! Pray I don't do anything too crazy this week!

Wednesday, June 27, 2007

My quest to catch a wave has lead me to this. I'm already a little goofy, but I have to be goofy-footed. That basically means standing on the board with the right foot (not the left foot) forward. I usually stand with the left foot forward so this will be a big adjustment! Luckily I'm still fairly new to the sport so it shouldn't affect me that much. I'm going to the beach again this weekend to try it out.

I've been home alone for the first time in about a year and a half! It's been great. I've been more productive with the new "projects" I'm starting (stay tuned), but I'm also finding out how difficult some things are:

1. **I tried making eggs for breakfast (good thing I like them scrambled... the ataxia in my left hand doesn't help.)**
2. **It took me a little over 30 mins to get the mail with the walker (a ~500-foot walk with doors to unlock, uneven pavement, and 6 steps up and 6 steps down one way.) It was the first time I did it by myself.**
3. **Cleaning my bathtub on my own. (I was visualizing Mr. Miagi telling me to *wax on* and *wax off*.)**

4. **Relying on other people for transportation is still the toughest thing to deal with (car=independence/social life.)**

Overall I think my time alone went pretty well. It's the closet thing I've had to a "vacation" in a year and a half. Can't wait until it's permanent.

Friday, July 6, 2007

I've always liked the martial arts. I took tae kwon do when I was a kid because I wanted to learn how to punch, kick, and break boards. I credit it for teaching me discipline at a very young age. My newfound enjoyment of reading has lead me to tai chi, a less violent form of martial arts. I started looking into alternative or complementary therapies out of curiosity. A friend has helped me discover yoga and introduced me to the mind-body concept of healing. Initially I thought it was a load of crap, but there are actually a lot of articles about that stuff in respected research journals. Tai chi has been studied numerous times in the elderly population for stress reduction and balance training. To my knowledge it hasn't been looked at in the brain tumor or young adult population. There are many survivors that could benefit from reduced stress, improved balance, physical activity, or even social interaction. hmmmm...

Something else I've stumbled upon is www.clinicaltrials.gov. This is a great way for patients to access the latest experimental treatments/medications. Joining a study will let the participant contribute to the fight against a certain disease and doing so can sometimes give complimentary healthcare follow-ups to participants. This is a great way to get care if you can't afford it. The catch is that the treatments/medicines are untested. They could either work out really well or you could get complications. It's a gamble, but you can make an informed decision and less of a gamble thanks to the Internet. Talk to your doctor before getting in a study.

Wednesday, July 11, 2007

Well, I had another book signing/lecture tonight. Turnout was twice as big as the last one. I think my next event will be even bigger. I'm actually getting more comfortable speaking in front of large crowds. Things went pretty smoothly except for a brief incident where my "allergies" got the best of me. I'm usually a pretty stoic guy, but whenever I hit a certain part of the presentation, my voice starts to crack which leads to leaky eyes. I'm sure this will pass. No more events until September so I can just focus on getting better and work on fixing my "allergies." One more down. Thanks to everyone that showed up.

Monday, July 16, 2007

July 14... just another day. Bastille Day maybe, but my birthday not that big a deal. Spent the weekend at the beach. I still haven't stood up yet. I'm so close! I need a little help paddling out, but I will stand by the end of the summer! Thanks to everyone that is helping me do this. That's all I want for my birthday. Screw the gifts and cake. Those things only last an instant. Accomplishing and doing what you want is something that you will enjoy forever. I'm so close!

Wednesday, July 17, 2007

Jus sanguinis... Latin for the "Right of Blood." My mother is a Canadian citizen and a legal resident alien of the United States. Maybe I should apply for dual American-Canadian Citizenship...I just saw the Michael Moore film "Sicko." Of course things were sensationalized, but for me it did bring a lot of issues to the surface. Here in America many people don't have access to good healthcare.

As stated by Thomas Jefferson in the Declaration of Independence, every American has the right to life, liberty, and the pursuit of happiness. Unfortunately, competition and the pursuit of money in the health"care" industry take away some of these rights. I do agree with Moore that some people suffer when insurance companies deny claims, pinch pennies, and make their CEOs richer. Is socialized medicine the answer to America's health "care" crisis? America is one of the richest countries in the world, but our health "care" system is more of a health "business." Let's face it, there is no easy solution until health "care" focuses on the patient again.

We've become a society that wants a quick fix to everything. Medications do help, but should be used as an adjunct treatment to education, prevention, health maintenance, and an active lifestyle. Our wealth as a country has made us obese and lazy. I think when we are young we need to reassess our health practices. We need to realize that while there may be a quick fix to a problem via medication, we need to address the root of the problem.

Do Canadian Citizens have it easier in terms of socialized healthcare? This will also require more investigation.

Thursday, July 26, 2007

Young people with cancer or other devastating diagnoses are a patient population that is getting stronger. I personally am tired of hearing "Oh you're young, you should do fine." This may be true, but many young adults aren't so lucky. I've had the pleasure of meeting a few young adults addressing situations more difficult than mine and observing how they handle their situation. They are the people who inspire me. Organizations like <u>I'm Too Young For This</u>, <u>Planet Cancer</u>, and <u>LIVESTRONG Young Adult Alliance</u> do a great job providing support for adolescents and young adults facing a scary cancer diagnosis. Since there is no cure yet for cancer, survivorship support is essential. I relied on my friends and family for this support. I am very lucky to have a strong network around me. I applaud these aforementioned organizations for their efforts because it is tough enough being a young adult. As a young adult, you are faced with these common dilemmas:

1. **Establishing your independence**
2. **Finding that special someone/starting your own family**
3. **Accomplishing your personal goals**

4. **Following your professional goals**
5. **Enjoying your youth**

Cancer or some other devastating diagnosis definitely doesn't make things any easier. Priorities change. I'm still in the process of "reinventing" myself. I'm still the same guy I was before, but I'm much more aware of different issues around me. I feel like I've aged 20 years since everything happened.

I'd like to announce the "Tumors Suck!" group on Facebook the new social networking platform young people are using more frequently. I've recruited a few other young adults to help me with this project. It should be an exciting undertaking! Join <u>Facebook</u> and join the "Tumors Suck!" group!

Sunday, July 29, 2007

Surfing attempt #5. Got to my feet, but for only for maybe 2 seconds. I did get out to the line up with some help, of course. Now I just want to sit and chill on a board. That has always been the fun part of surfing for me. Thanks to everyone who have helped me out. The goals now are to stand for at least 5 seconds, paddle out myself, and sit and turn quick enough to paddle and catch a wave. SOOOO close! I did a few face plants onto the board, so I got a couple cuts and bumps on my face. I think that they actually look cool! I have a couple new ideas how I can "remedy" these issues, but I bet I'm tiring everyone out. So props to them on taking baby steps with me! Don't laugh! Harry Potter is calling me!

Tuesday, August 7, 2007

I think it's time to get behind the wheel again. I'm starting to get tired of relying on people if I want to go somewhere. I appreciate all their help, but I feel like such a mooch. I have managed to talk people into letting me drive in empty parking lots… hee hee. I should be looking into the legal way of doing this. I never realized this before, but for me driving represents independence and a social life again. Anyone have suggestions?

Sunday, August 12, 2007

I'm starting to find out there is a lot I can do on my own… I took a train up to LA from SD by myself this weekend to hangout with some old and new friends. Before I start into that, big props go to my friends for putting up with me for the weekend, taking me to the *Bourne Ultimatum*, for gracing me with their presence at the I2Y meet-up in LA, for splitting dim sum, and for the awesome bbq in Santa Monica!

Anyways, growing up in the Midwest and living in California, no one ever takes the train. The stations are so cool here in CA because they have a 1930's feel to them. I always feel like I should be wearing a fedora in there. Anyways, I got to LA on Friday night and went straight to the bar to meet up with the LA I2Y crew. Really cool peeps! We all share a common goal to increase awareness for 15-39 year olds dealing with cancer and other crap! I had myself a nice cold beer and a smile the rest of the night… Alcohol hits me a lot faster than it used to… which isn't saying much. I'd forgotten how beautiful the women in LA are and how much I stick out with my walker. It is really fun meeting other people like myself who want to make a difference.

Sat… slept in and went to Chinese dim sum with some old friends. Dude, for those you who have never heard of dim sum, it's kind of like a buffet where you don't have to move! Sweet! Basically, they bring carts of food to you and you decide then and there if you want to eat it. You can point to what you want or wave them away. But the catch is you have to pay by plate and most of the time I never know what I'm eating. I just eat it first and then decide if I like it or not. You can tell me how "exotic" it is after I eat it. It has to pass the "inspection" first. It's automatically ruled out if it still has eyes, smells weird, or if too many people are watching me eat it to see my reaction. The colors green or yellow usually are "red flags," but if they pass smell and eye ball test, then I'll try it. "Galvez tested and approved" We ate a lot… enough to put me in food coma. Caught a movie and got back in time for a BBQ. Caribbean rum and beer ended my palate-friendly day.

Sunday went to *IHOP*. The Stuffed French Toast combo is now my favorite thing there. As we were driving to *IHOP*, I remembered how much I hate LA traffic and how crowded it is there! I felt ready to go back to good ole laid-back and sunny San Diego, my new "home!" Then I was able to take a nap on the choo-choo train back to SD.

Sunday, August 19, 2007

Let me premise this entry by saying I have never willingly watched *Dancing with the Stars!* I'm not disrespecting it because it takes a lot of talent to do what they do. I just prefer watching competitions where the scoring is consistent and not dependent on judges. I digress... So anyways the last two times I've gone out, we've gone to places with music I'm into. I'm getting out more and picking up where I left off in 2005. I've noticed that my rhythm is slowly coming back. I'm no Usher or Justin Timberlake, but I can now feel a beat and respond somewhat rhythmically. First it was the head bob. Now it's the shoulder shrugs. My rhythm is slowly returning, moving down my body. Once I get my hips and legs back... oh boy... look out!

Will be looking into the driving program at Sharp Memorial. Getting behind the wheel is the next major step.

I've been doing workouts on my own at my complex's pool. Walking in the water, swimming, and trying to run in place... totally wipes me out. Need a little patience...

Thursday, September 6, 2007

This weekend I was back in the Midwest for the first time in a long time. I miss the green and foliage in Michigan. I'll be back in MI for a month in the fall. It will be my "home base" for my fall book tour.

Anyways, I'm trying to figure out how to keep myself busy on my down time in the Midwest. I figured apple picking will be perfect for dynamic standing balance and coordination. Plus apple orchards in the fall are the best! The smells, the fresh donuts, the warm apple cider, the pies, the colors, aahhhh...

Anyways, this past weekend was great. I had the pleasure of attending a wedding of a good friend and hanging out with some people I haven't seen in a while. I got in a couple days before the wedding and convinced my dad to let me drive around the neighborhood. Hahaha! More of that is planned when I'm home again. I think I'm more mischievous now than I when I was a kid.

Took a road trip to the wedding outside of Chicago. The wedding was beautiful and I had so much fun being with my friends. I even made it out to the dance floor for a slow song and another song. I think I'm OK out there if I have a partner to hold on to/hold on to me. I was lucky enough to find someone brave enough to take that risk with me. It was fun, but I hate asking for help with the simplest things. I can't wait until this is over. When I have "liquid courage" in me, I'm more apt to trying the things I think I should be doing. The intelligent, cautious professional in me loosens up. I was able to make it to the dance floor without the cane (with some help of course), walk down 2 flights of steps, and practice walking by myself around empty tables. I was so pooped when I finally got back home to San Diego. I have 2 more weekends to go surfing. I still have a lot of stuff planned this fall... hee hee (there is more stuff in the works)... stay tuned!

Tuesday, September 11, 2007

My name is Eric and I'm addicted to football. (Hi, Eric.) I did absolutely nothing but watch TV this weekend. I watched my beloved Wolverines drop to levels I've never seen, watched my fantasy football teams "compete," and watched my Lions open with a dramatic win. This fall is going to be busy, so I will take any opportunity to be a football sloth. I'm heading back to Michigan for a month to kick off my book tour. So much traveling coming up, I hope I'm ready for everything planned. The mind is willing, but I'm not sure how my body will hold up. It seems like I need a "siesta" everyday. Oh well, I'll figure out how to pull this off.

Monday, September 17, 2007

Things are really starting to get busy! My cousin from Toronto is in town. She is my not-so-baby cousin now. She cracks me up. Anyways, took her to my new favorite cheap sushi place in SD, and my mom took her shopping. We went to the beach and she watched me wipe out. (Caught a few on my knees but standing on the board is giving me fits... I'll get it next summer!) She also came to a few doctor appointments with me and we went out to eat a number of times. All that on top of getting a press release ready for my fall book tour (I'm still surprised at everything I've pulled off thus far!), a brain tumor conference, my other projects, and getting my personal affairs ready for my extended trip.

The conference was very informational and I was able to meet some really cool people there. It was my first brain tumor-related conference. I got to rub elbows with some of the directors of the National Brain Tumor Foundation, the chair for meningioma research at UCSF, and most importantly other brain tumor survivors and loved ones of survivors. I also got to learn a little about stereotactic radiosurgery. As I suspected, I was one of the younger attendees. I very easily found other young adults in the room and we all subconsciously congregated in the same area. Watching each presentation made me feel like I was in school again. I followed everything, but I looked around the room and some of the faces surrounding me were marked with blank stares. Being around other people that had to deal with "crap" was actually kind of cool. For the first time in a long time, I didn't feel completely alone. Of course I stuck out because of the walker (I still don't have the guts to go out by myself with the cane) and my trusty baseball cap, but I didn't feel out of place there.

My time screwing around has passed, so now it's time to kick it into the next gear! The next couple months are going to be crazy. Stay tuned... don't be surprised at some of the stuff I have in the works! I'll try to update the blog as much as I can... it's gonna be a busy fall. =D hee hee

My summer was a time for myself, but I was starting to sail into unchartered waters. The fall would not only be the start of book tour, but I would also launch a few new projects. I can't seem to sit still. I haven't had a break since the surgery. Returning to the life I once knew was my only objective. I was getting more involved with young survivor organizations and brain tumor organizations. Is a new direction in life starting to reveal itself? The book tour would help me realize that I can still help people, but is this what I want to do?

# Stronger

Th-th-that that don't kill me
Can only make me stronger
I need you to hurry up now
Cause I can't wait much longer

**-Kanye West,** *Graduation* 2007

I did more traveling in the fall of 2007 than I had in a long time. My first book tour was a lot of fun. It stopped in Evanston, IL; Flint, MI; Oakland, CA; and New York, NY. I didn't realize how many people I knew in different parts of the country! I had friends to catch up with everywhere I went. I also learned some very interesting facts about brain tumors and young adult survivors. Those facts drew me into the world of advocacy. It is hard work! The Facebook Tumors Suck and my new mAss Kickers group were getting a lot of hits. I was starting to rub elbows with the major players in the young adult survivor and brain tumor community.

Wednesday, September 26, 2007

Well, I got into Michigan last Wednesday. Had a bachelor party to go to on Friday. We got a suite at Comerica Park to watch the Detroit Tigers play the KC Royals. There were 19 guys that showed up. So much fun seeing old friends and watching our childhood team compete for the wild card playoff spot. We went to the casino afterwards, but unfortunately it was too crowded to get a spot for all of us at the craps table. All good though cause I got to catch up with some friends I haven't seen in a really long time. It was the first time some of my friends have seen me since the surgery. I wonder what they were thinking.

Part 2 of the bachelor party was "the classic," which is basically a day of sports competitions highlighted by a double elimination 2-on-

2 basketball tournament and a 4-on-4 backyard football playoff. The theme for the classic this year was "Bling." Hilarious! Little John "pimp cups" were distributed as trophies and people came dressed up in "thug gear." It was so hard watching from the sideline as my friends competed for the coveted pimp cups. I'm so used to being in the thick of things when it comes to sports. It sucked realizing that I can't do the things I love doing. It was a harsh reminder that things are different now, and it has made me more hungry to get what I want. My priorities are different now, but my spirit is far from broken. Everyday I learn something new about myself. I continue to test my limits. I think that this makes me stronger because I'm always reassessing everything that happened... the "good" and the "bad."

This weekend I go to Northwestern University in Evanston, IL on my first stop of my book tour. Part of me still can't believe I pulled this off! I will be going public with my new projects very soon... stay tuned!


Monday, October 1, 2007

Man, it was a busy weekend! Went to Chicago with a few friends from PT school. I also had my first stop on my "book tour" at Northwestern University. I still refer to it as my "book tour" because it's just a good reason to hangout with my friends in different parts of the country. Chicago is beautiful. If I were to live in the Midwest, there is no doubt in my mind I would be in Chicago.

Anyways, I stayed in Wrigleyville. A friend of mine lives a block from Wrigley Field, where the Chicago Cubs play. It's a bustling part of town. I love the fact that you can walk everywhere and it is so green there. I miss the green/fall colors of the Midwest. I think I would eventually like to settle down in the Midwest. All my friends are getting married or in serious relationships. I'm one of the last bachelors. No one really addresses this, but being a young, single survivor and dating is a tough order to fill. First off you worry about your physical appearance to others. How will "potentials" be attracted to you? Then you worry about being able to fulfill/perform traditional male/female "activities." Hahaha… you know what I mean. Yeah I'll go there! All I know is that I feel like I'm in Jr. High again. I think I'm just a little "cooler." A little… I could go on, but I digress.

Saturday was the Michigan-Northwestern game. I've now seen the Wolverines play at the Big House, the Rose Bowl, the Horseshoe, Spartan Stadium, and Ryan Stadium at NU. Took the wheelchair with us for the sake of time. I really hate that thing, but it is still necessary for long distances. Because of the chair, we got prime seats in the first row behind the end-zone. You could actually see the facial expressions on the players' faces. Great seats! We took the train to Evanston. There is no way I could have been quick enough with the cane to deal with the crowds getting to the stadium and the train.

Sunday was my first stop on my "book tour" at Northwestern sponsored by Lambda Phi Epsilon and Kaibigan (the Filipino-American Association at NU.) I really enjoyed it. It was great to watch Kaibigan perform the *tinikling*. Took me back to undergrad and performing with FASA (the Filipino American Student Association) at U of M with my friends. I really enjoyed seeing the bros of Lambda Phi Epsilon. 10 years ago, I was one of the pledge dads for their founding fathers. It is so cool to see how everything has grown and evolved. It's nice to see that the same principles and characteristics on which we were founded are still evident in the current bros.

I like to think college was a pivotal time in my life and really shaped who I am today. I was raised in Ann Arbor, but grew up at the University of Michigan. I learned to be a leader through Lambda Phi Epsilon. I learned where I came from through FASA. I'm still trying to figure out the next step. I have an idea. Check out my latest project. www.masskickers.com. Details to follow. Oh yeah, **save 10/25 in your calendar for the inagural "**Tumors Suck**" Day**. Wear a shirt or drink from a mug out in public to spread awareness for the plight of young adults 15-39 dealing with some serious health issues. More stuff is in the works… Stay tuned!

Sunday, October 7, 2007

Friday I had another event at my old grad school stomping grounds in Flint, MI. There was a great turnout. Many of my old friends from PT school were there. Some of my friends from undergrad were there, as well. A friend from high school was there, too! It was great to see everyone. The event went pretty well. My "allergies" still bother me whenever I hit a certain part of the presentation. I don't think it has gotten any easier. I'm usually a pretty stoic guy. I hate that part. Anyways, other than my "allergy attack" things went well. I fielded some great questions from my PT colleagues. I think people are starting to take notice and understand the plight of brain tumor patients and young adult survivors!

I'm at the halfway point of my tour, but I still have a few things to do in MI. I get a few days in San Diego at the end of the month then I'm off to Oakland, CA. After that it's to NY. Things are starting to get serious. Dude, I hope I know what I'm getting myself into…

Sunday, October 14, 2007

This was the first weekend in a while where I didn't have anything "official" scheduled. I think I have adult ADD… so I found ways to keep myself busy. On Friday, I met up with some friends from high school for a drink. Was really cool catching up with everyone. I hadn't seen a lot of them since graduation. Many of them are married with children. I wonder how different my life would be if I stayed in Michigan. Those thoughts quickly leave my head as fast as an offensive lineman moves in an all-you-can-eat buffet. I have no regrets about anything I've done. I've always done what I need to do, then move on. Anyways, I realized that in high school I thought I knew what I wanted to do when I "grow up." This whole brain tumor experience has opened a lot of doors, now I have to figure out what my next move is. All I know is I still want to remain in the health "care" field… putting the "care" back in healthcare.

Saturday, I went to the apple orchard with my mom and her friends. Fall is my favorite time of the year in the Midwest. The colors, the smells, and cool crisp air can't be found in my new home in San Diego. The experience of eating fresh cider mill donuts is unparalleled. Man, the smells bring back so many pleasant memories of wearing a sweatshirt to stay warm, but taking it off and tying it around my waist cause the sun made it too hot to wear. The cool breeze, warm sun, and crisp air always made your skin grateful you took off your sweatshirt.

Later that evening my friend picked me up and we met up with some of his wife's friends at a vegetarian restaurant. I've never been to a vegetarian restaurant before so I didn't know what to expect. I was surprisingly full when I left. I played it safe and got a sandwich, but I was eyeing someone's ravioli the whole time. After the restaurant we hit up some bar. The thing is… I still need someone to hold my arm if I go out and use the cane. If I use the walker, I'm slow as molasses but at least I'm independent. I can't wait to get rid of that thing! I only use the cane when I go out if I trust that the people with whom I'm going out will safely walk with me. I'm going to Canada tomorrow on an unscheduled trip for a few days. I've got to write my speech for a wedding next weekend. Back to business.


Tuesday, October 23, 2007

It was a crazy week! I can't believe 6 weeks have already passed! On Monday I took an impromptu trip to Toronto. I got to see so many of my relatives there. I also got to visit my grandmother's grave. It was the first time I visited her since the funeral in 2003. So much has happened since then. Standing there in front of her grave reminded me of how precious life is and how we need to enjoy every moment of it. Spending time with my relatives was great! But I'm always a little leery whenever my mom and my aunts get together. I always feel like they are scheming to set me up with someone. I hate that!

Thursday was the rehearsal/rehearsal dinner for the wedding. I really wanted to use the cane for the ceremony, but I'm still not confident enough yet to use the cane by myself. My brother and my dad think that I'm not focusing on my rehab enough. They may be right. I've got to get back to focusing on myself. I have a lot on my plate right now, but part of me likes being busy. If I have learned anything from being a physical therapist, I should know how to take care of myself. There is very strong potential that I will get carried away with all my "projects." I can be a little obsessive compulsive when I'm really into something. Ask my old roommates about my Nintendo-Zelda marathons. That is why I never got into Playstation/Xbox. My OCD would have kept me in front of the TV for hours.

Anyways, the wedding was great! So many people were there. I actually had to give a best man speech in front of 270 people. I'm getting more comfortable speaking in front of people, but I still don't like it. Apparently I'm pretty good at making people cry. Hee hee… I guess that's a good thing. My next stop on the tour is in Oakland, CA at Samuel Merritt College. I'll get to see more friends from the Bay area, my godson, some cousins and hopefully my new nephew. I'm excited! I was supposed to fly back to San Diego today, but with all the craziness down there right now, I decided to fly directly to San Francisco from Michigan on Saturday. Some of my friends have lost their homes to the wildfires. My thoughts and prayers are with them.

Thursday, October 25, 2007 TUMORS SUCK DAY

Two years ago today my life took an unexpected turn. I'm now following a new path. I didn't choose this path. It chose me. That tumor picked the wrong guy to mess with! Help me spread awareness. Today is Tumors Suck Day, but spreading awareness doesn't have to be limited to just today. COPY AND PASTE THE BELOW TEXT AND PUT IT ON YOUR BLOG OR EMAIL ALL YOUR CONTACTS!

************

**-70,000 people ages 15-39 are diagnosed with cancer each year**
**-Young adults with cancer have a lower survival rates with respect to the geriatric and pediatric populations.**

**-There is little research on young adults aged 15-39 to combat this disturbing fact.**

Why don't people know about this? Help me spread awareness. As a brain tumor survivor, I now understand how scary it is to hear those words "We found a tumor in your _____ (insert important body organ here)."

Wear a shirt or drink from a mug from here.

http://www.cafepress.com/tumorssuck

If you don't pick up an item from the shop to show support for TUMORS SUCK DAY, at least send out a copy of this message to all your friends. The goal of this day is to raise awareness for young adults dealing with some serious health issues.

TUMORS SUCK! KEEP FIGHTING!

-Eric AKA "Galvez"


Monday, November 5, 2007

Whew... So far this fall has been a blur! Shoot... the past 2 years have been a blur! I have a few days in San Diego before I hit the road again. Just got back from L.A. to see my friends get married. It was a beautiful Hindu wedding. The food and hotel were amazing! Both the bride and groom looked astonishing in their traditional wedding clothes. The coolest part of the ceremony was the fact that the groom rode in on a horse! I'm so glad I got to witness the whole extravaganza. I really enjoy experiencing other cultures.

I got back from Michigan last week and had 2 days in San Diego before my 3rd stop on the tour at Samuel Merritt College in Oakland, CA. I stayed with a friend of mine and his family. Got a taste of family life, and decided that is for me someday. After attending so many weddings of close friends you can't help but think of the next step in life. I guess the first step for me is finding a girlfriend. hahaha! Being a younger single guy recovering from a brain tumor doesn't make things any easier. Right now my eyes are focused on getting back on my feet...

literally. I have way too many projects coming up to concern myself with this stuff. That's my excuse and I'm sticking to it. Next week I go to New York. No lecture is scheduled, but I do have a stop scheduled at the NYU Hassenfeld Pediatric cancer center. It has been fun catching up with friends, but all this traveling is making me pooped!

Monday, November 12, 2007

I've been doing some random reading lately. I read something about *the Stockdale Paradox*. It basically describes the attitude to have in order to overcome adversity. In a nutshell you have to *remain positive, while at the same time be wary of the reality/facts of the situation*. Lean too heavily on one side and you set yourself up for disappointment or lean too heavily on the other side and you psyche yourself out. Finding balance to this paradox is the key! Pretty random reading, but an interesting read nonetheless. I've never really been into reading, but now it seems like I am finding a new hobby. TV just isn't appealing anymore. Except for sporting events. Sports has all the ingredients: action, drama, emotion, suspense, cheerleaders… what more do you need? Hahaha! There are a few shows I like, but reality TV and game shows have turned me against primetime TV.

Anyways, I had 3 days in San Diego before I took another unscheduled trip to L.A. One of my friends and his family were visiting L.A. for the extended weekend. I jumped at the chance to hangout with them! I took the train from San Diego again… it is getting easier to travel by myself because at least I know what to expect. I do need help though. The attendants at the train station are really helpful. They have this thing called the "Red Cap" service to assist people getting to the train, plus they actually talk to you like a regular person.

While I was in LA I visited one of my friends in Westwood. He lives on a pretty steep hill with 6 tall entrance steps and no hand rail to enter the house. It was a challenge just getting from the car into the house with the walker, but I did it. After hanging out a few hours, I had to repeat this challenge in reverse. I was not so successful. While my friends were saying goodbye to each other, I decided to wait for them outside with the walker on the steps. Not a good idea. I lost my balance and tumbled down 6 steps onto the hill. A small bush halted my unexpected descent down the hill. Actually, my right foot ended up in the bush. It all happened so fast, but it felt like slow motion as it was happening. As soon as I hit the ground I did a quick assessment of everything, no pain and nothing broken but my ego. I looked up at the top of the stairs and saw my 2 friends staring at me with their mouths wide open! I found this really funny for some reason so I couldn't help but laugh a little. Well, they helped me up to my feet and back into the car. I'm a little weird because I was laughing about the whole incident on the car ride back to my friend's place. That walker is stable but not very maneuverable. I think it actually contributed to my tumble down the stairs. I can't wait to get rid of it! I'm really lucky I walked away from that fall with only a few scrapes. If I was older, I could have seriously hurt myself.

Anyways it was a fun weekend. I have 2 days in San Diego then I'm in New York for a week for the last stop on my tour. Maybe I can relax when I get back from New York… Maybe…


Wednesday, November 21, 2007

Whew! The book tour is over and I'm exhausted, but I have a few new ideas I've picked up along the way… hee hee hee. Once I catch my breath things will start to roll again. I'm seriously learning a lot about myself. I'm doing a lot of things I never dreamed I would do. Raising money for charity, writing a book, going on a book tour, public speaking, and some other stuff in the works…

Anyways, my last and final stop was in New York. I didn't realize how many friends I have there. The people I used to watch *Saved By The Bell* reruns and go to the bar with are now investment bankers, architects, university employees, graphic designers, lawyers, and medical professionals. Who would have thought!

I got in on Wednesday night. On Thursday my Ninang (Filipino Godmother) wanted to throw a cocktail party for me. I've never been to a cocktail party before. Pretty good turnout. On Friday I spent some time in Jersey with family. My little baby cousins aren't babies anymore! On Saturday, watched the GAME and was disappointed once again. I applaud all of Coach Carr's accomplishments. He will go down in Michigan football history as the classiest coach to lead the Wolverines. It takes a big man to know when to step aside. Saturday night I went to a swanky engagement party at the top of some hotel in Manhattan. Sunday I met with a young adult brain tumor survivor in physical therapy school at NYU for lunch. Later I had dinner with Matthew Zachary, the executive director of *I'm Too Young For This*. I may be getting more involved with them.

But to top it all off… I was invited to the young adult support group at the *NYU Hassenfeld Pediatric Cancer Center*. I've never been to a live support group before so I had no idea what to expect. They had me at "free pizza." But seriously, it was cool to see how these guys bounce back. I really felt a bond with them. I was the oldest one in the room for a change.

I need a few days to recover. I don't want to wear myself out, but there is a lot that needs to be done. Join the facebook "Tumors Suck" group to get an idea of what I've got planned…

Saturday, November 24, 2007

As the power of the Internet provides more information about one's new diagnosis, the need for a consolidated strictly information site for the newly diagnosed patient and their loved ones has emerged. Patients are continually looking for information online. mAss Kickers will fulfill this need by offering links to diagnosis-specific organizations, informational books by leading experts, and inspirational books by survivors of specific diagnoses to provide knowledge, courage, and strength through this intimidating process. mAss Kickers is a unique website because it:

- **Promotes courage for patients and their loved ones through unity and a fighting attitude**
- **Offers support for the newly-diagnosed patient, current patients, loved ones of patients, and survivors via a unique diagnosis-specific discussion board**
- **Empowers patients and more importantly the newly-diagnosed patient through knowledge**
- **Offers diagnosis-specific books for purchase written by leading experts and inspirational survivors**
- **Offers links to diagnosis specific organizations**
- **Fundraises for research in diagnosis-specific organizations**

As a brain tumor survivor I realize how scary and intimidating a new diagnosis can be. My purpose for spear-heading the creation of this web site is to empower patients through knowledge and to make patients feel less helpless when faced with an intimidating diagnosis. Just know that you are not alone.

ARE YOU A MASS KICKER?
The site is coming soon! Keep an eye out for it. Spread the word.

Tuesday, December 4, 2007

I always find a way to keep myself busy. If I have an opportunity to do something I'll figure out how I can do it... 1) if it's practical or 2) if I really want to do it. You have to have a very logical argument against me or I'll do it anyways. This whole week I was exhausted, but I really wanted to go up to L.A. on Friday for the *Stupid Cancer Happy Hour* sponsored by **I'm Too Young For This**. People were telling me to slow down and take a break, but I really wanted to show my support for young adult survivors because I now realize how unique we are from other "survivors." Very few people understand what we've been through. We were all doing our thing, trying to establish ourselves... then BOOM... our lives get interrupted by some devastating diagnosis.

Then we scramble to get back on track. Some of us get back faster than others, but we all go through similar crap. I've found that most of the survivors I've met have a new found passion for something. I guess a brush with your own mortality refocuses priorities. So anyways, I'm glad I went because I got to hangout with other mAss Kickers closer to my age. There were some great live performances by young adult survivor musicians and I finally got to hangout with some people that understand firsthand what I've been through.

I came back to San Diego the next day and took some friends around the area. I showed them La Jolla, Sea World, and Balboa Park. I discovered a few new things at Sea World! Read... Anheuser-Bush Hospitality Center with free beer samples. I'm definitely making a stop there next time. I also introduced my friends to the "California" Burrito (available only in San Diego). OK... Now it's time to REST before going back to Michigan for the holidays.


Wednesday, December 19, 2007

Dude! I definitely have lost my cold tolerance. I'm now what my friends from PT school call "Candy." It's really cold in Michigan! It's so nice to see snow, but a few days of it is good enough. I'm here for two weeks. This year I'm going to a "'89 Prom" themed New Year's party. It's going to be hilarious! I hope I can find my old neon sunglasses.

Surprisingly, I've been doing a lot of reading lately. The TV has been turned off and the warm spot on the carpet next to the heating vent has become my favorite spot in the room. The "nerd" in me is reborn. I'm currently reading some book called *Genome: The autobiography of a species in 23 chapters*. It's like reading a textbook with a story. This would be pretty dry reading for most people, but as a biology major it was neat seeing names I recognize like Watson, Crick, and Gregor Mendel. What was even cooler was reading their personal stories... stuff you never hear about in the classroom. Watson was only in his 30s when he made the groundbreaking discovery of DNA! It's crazy knowing that huge leaps in mankind can be made now that we know more about our "blueprint" from the *Human Genome Project*. I don't think people realize the importance of this discovery.

Anyways, I have a busy trip planned in Michigan. This weekend I'll be meeting up with some friends from PT school, then meeting up with some high school friends. This website has really connected me with a lot of people from my past: Friends from high school, college friends, old teachers, old coaches, and even new friends who understand/empathize with everything I've been through. Just connecting with people has already made writing the book worth all the effort. Much is planned in 2008… I can't wait to unveil it!


Wednesday, December 26, 2007

It seems like my weekends are always packed. This weekend was no different, especially because Christmas was right around the corner. On Friday night, I hung out with some friends from grad school in Ann Arbor. We are a crew of immature jokesters, which is why we get along so well. I also found out some of my friends are expecting their first little one this summer! Whoa… Congrats!

On Saturday night I went up to the Lansing area to hangout with some more friends and see my old roommate's new house. Jeez… all my friends have "grown up!" I've always been a late bloomer.

On Sunday my friend drove me back to Ann Arbor so I could meet up with some friends to watch some football. It wasn't exactly what I expected. It was like a mini high school reunion. So many familiar faces were there. People brought their significant others and kids! I was amazed because I was just expecting to watch some football. I didn't get to eat my BBQ Chicken Sandwich until I left because I was too busy catching up with everyone. I missed the 10-year reunion. A lot of my old teammates from football and wrestling were there. It was great because we just laughed at each other and relived old memories the whole time. The football and wrestling teams my senior year were tight like family. I hadn't seen many of these guys in almost 15 years! I still try to apply our team mottos in everything I do. "Count on me." "110%

No Excuses!" It was really great seeing everyone and look forward to the next gathering.

On Christmas Eve I met up with the family for dinner at some steakhouse and later church. I found out I walk faster without the cane, but I need at least one person (someone I trust) to hold my arm.

On Christmas Day we went to my Uncle's house for our traditional Christmas activities of lunch, 2 rounds of Feisty White Elephant, CCB (Corny Commentary Bingo), and dinner. The get-together is always huge! 5 families plus significant others... at least 20 people. A small family Christmas seems odd to me. I wonder how new significant others view this whole extravaganza. I was introduced to Guitar Hero! Fun and could be good to work on my left hand coordination... hmmmmm.

My trips are always packed. I don't mind because I've never felt alone since everything happened 2 years ago. I hit the next gear in 2008... Stay Tuned!


Monday, December 31, 2007

I guess this is the time everyone reflects on all that has happened over the year. 2007 was a very busy year. I welcome the potential that comes with 2008.

I set some goals and fell short (most notably with the return to running and the return to work as a physical therapist) but I still haven't given up on it yet. I've managed to adapt and accomplished a few things along the way: I published a book, got interviewed a few times, created Tumors Suck! Day, wrote a couple articles, went on a national book tour, attended a few weddings, and most importantly connected and reconnected with so many people. I definitely don't take things for granted anymore. I'm just happy to be around to enjoy the company of ALL my family and friends. A new year always brings hope and potential. I am very excited for 2008. I do have a lot up my sleeve the next few months. I think 2008 has the potential to be bigger than 2007 for me! Right now, that is all it is... potential. Once that potential becomes reality... Look out!

Now that the book tour was over and the New Year was starting, I was starting to realize that maybe I have a larger calling. While I was gaining more attention for what I was doing I still have the people closest to me reminding me that I shouldn't neglect my rehab. With the year came new expectations and goals. Re-establishing my independence was the hardest thing to do when surrounded by loved ones. Things were continuing to unfold. I found myself getting involved in things I knew very little about. In the coming months, I would learn how to balance high expectations for myself verses the stark reality of a situation. Many doors were opening up for me.

# Mr. Brightside

I'm coming out of my cage
And I'm doing just fine
Gotta gotta be down
Because I want it all.

**-The Killers,** *Hot Fuss* 2004

T hings were finally starting to look up. I had seen the "light at the end of the tunnel" for quite some time. I was finally starting to hear some birds on the outside. I realized I am even closer to getting out of that dark tunnel.

Thursday, January 10, 2008

Man, I think I'm coming down with something. I'm trying some new medication to help with the tremors in my right hand. Nothing has worked so far. While my mobility has been improving, I think I've been neglecting the fine motor ability in my hands. I've never liked taking medicine, but I'm at the point where I need to try every avenue. Medication is not cheap and usually has side effects. People think the Canadians have it all figured out with socialized medicine. I think it can work if you're in a demographic that doesn't immediately need it.

Clearly the American system has shortcomings as does the Canadian system. I do realize that there is no easy answer to the healthcare crisis. As technology creates more (efficient but expensive) treatments for devastating diagnoses, we will be trapped in the vicious circle of "should everyone have the right to healthcare… if so how do we regulate it?… if not how do people get healthcare?" Maybe some sort of "hybrid socialized private pay" system should be created.

I will be listening intently to see how the presidential candidates address this.

**Monday, January 14, 2008**

Well, I got my first real taste of getting denied for coverage by my HMO today. I am trying different medications to control the tremors in my hands. I've never been a big fan of taking medication, but the tremors are getting to the point where eating what I want is starting to get hard. I was at the pharmacist and was denied at the counter. My neurologist wanted to increase the dose of the current medication I'm trying, so I needed to get a prescription filled to get a stronger dose. Prior to that I was taking samples, but apparently it wasn't strong enough. Now I am faced with the dilemma of testing new medication with stronger side effects or pursuing an appeal with the HMO to get coverage for the stronger dose of medication. I have decided to try the new medication until I get this other issue resolved. In 2 months I will be eligible for Medicare disability insurance. Whoa… I'll be on Medicare at 32! I must be pretty "messed up" to qualify for Medicare disability since it is not easy to get. Medicare is a federal health care program for the elderly and disabled. I've been pretty lucky that the HMO has covered all of my health care expenses thus far. Some people aren't so lucky. My eyes are definitely opening to issues with the health "care" industry. I'm expecting a lot more red tape and future snafus with Medicare.

**Wednesday, January 23, 2008**

Well, I finally got what I've been waiting so long for… independence at least for a little while. My family is on vacation for a month leaving me all alone! All this time I've constantly had someone with me telling me what to do or distracting me with encouragement that I appreciate tremendously. It's just nice to have some alone time. I've adjusted and learned to block people out. Simple tasks like going out to get the mail, cooking dinner, grocery shopping, going out with friends, etc. require a little extra time, preparation, and assistance since I can't drive yet.

Although I've been enjoying my time alone, I'm still pretty busy. Mark your calendars because I'm having a book signing at the Michigan

Union @ U of M in Ann Arbor 10/5/08. Coincidence that it is the same weekend as Homecoming weekend Michigan-Illinois? Hmmmm…. try to make it to A2 that weekend. It will be a great game! Oh yeah, I hear there is a really cool book signing the day after the game. More stuff is in the works, stay tuned…

Wednesday, January 30, 2008

Week two has been fun. I'm quickly realizing that in order for me to maintain my work "activities," exercise, and activities of daily living, something had to give if I am to live by myself. After some time alone, a good friend of mine spent a few days with me and helped me realize this. I've been so busy lately concentrating on my other projects that I have been neglecting my own recovery! The cavalier/fearless attitude that got me here is getting complacent. Just what I needed… a wake-up call! I will not be able to accomplish all my goals alone. Good Roommate=Good Workout Partner. I still have a long way to go. Can I get comfortable?… Yes. Did I accomplish what I wanted?… Nope. Wake-up call!

My friend took me to my follow up MRI. My third one since the surgery. Surprisingly, I wasn't nervous about it until I laid down on the table and they clamped my head into the harness. Before they put you in the MRI they give you ear plugs to block out the sounds around you. However, they don't block out everything. The earplugs actually AMPLIFY the sounds of your own heartbeat and breath rate. For people who get claustrophobic this may pose a problem. For me, once I focus on the wise words of Mr. Miagi, "In through nose. Out through mouth. In. Out." I'm so relaxed I'm practically asleep.

I picked up a CD of my MRI films in the same waiting room where I waited to get my first MRI. It kinda took me back to the place that would change my life forever. I just realized that the last time I was there, was the last time I felt like a "regular" person. My head was filed with anxiety after that 1st MRI waiting for the initial results. "Virgin pre-MRI Galvez" had no worries. "Deflowered-MRI Galvez" was a little worried something was up. This time around I took home a copy of the MRI on CD. Luckily, my friend visiting me is a physician so together we tried to interpret the MRI. Pretty funny cause earlier in the week we went grocery shopping. He is one of those guys where your maturity level drops when you hang out together. I don't know if it's me or if it's him, but we both act like grade-schoolers when left unattended. So anyways, we were walking down this aisle at the grocery store and this chubby "Super Mario"-looking guy with baggy jeans and no underwear stops about 3 feet in front of me and bends over to pick up a can of soup. He must have been reading all the nutritional info on the cans or something cause I was stuck there in my walker staring at 4 inches of butt crack for what seemed like an eternity! He got up pretty nonchalantly. No worries that he just shocked the living daylights out of two innocent bystanders. No apologies. No adjustments. As he was walking away, I bit my lip and tried to hold in my laughter. Then I heard my friend say something. I couldn't hold it in any longer and let the laugh escape from my mouth in a violent explosion from my lips! Then we both were cracking up. The cute girl on the cell phone was shaking her head in disapproval as we passed by.

On a more serious note, the MRI looked OK. No re-growth from what we could see. We have to wait and see what the radiologist says. I see the neurosurgeon next.


Thursday, February 7, 2008

Week Three has been great, but I'm starting to realize that being by myself isn't all it's cracked up to be. I've been fighting for my own independence this whole time, but by doing so I'm also inadvertently pushing people away. There has got to be some sort of balance or equilibrium point! That's the trick! Living by myself was fine when I could drive around and actually go places on my own. I feel like a prisoner in my own home. The Internet has become my best friend. I don't go out to work to see other people, only a handful of people come visit, I only get out so often to get the mail. I only get to see people when they want to see me. I hate not being able to go out and hangout with who I want, where I want, when I want. I was hardly ever at home before I found out about that tumor. It drives me nuts cause cognitively I'm fine, but physically I'm still not there yet! Thank God I have stuff keeping me "busy" cause, dude, I can see how one could easily fall into depression! Speaking of busy... I just found out I was selected to be a participant in the next *Head to Hollywood* Event and I am 1 of 4 recipients of the *SHARP Victories of Spirit Eagle Award*. More stuff in the works... stay tuned...

Wednesday, February 13, 2008

I think I just made a huge mistake. Ever since I graduated high school, I promised myself I would not start playing video games again because I tend to get a little obsessive compulsive. I had one lapse after graduating college playing the Legend of Zelda. Everyday, for about a month, I was in front of the TV for hours after work. I always liked those kind of games because of the story lines. I used to like playing those games just to see the ending. I am borrowing my dad's Nintendo Wii. I just got Guitar Hero III to... uhhhhh work on my fine motor control in my left hand. I can monitor my progress by looking at my score... an "objective" measure! It's actually kinda fitting because I used to listen to *Guns N Roses, Motley Crue, Bon Jovi*, and *Def Leppard* when I was a kid playing Super Mario Bros II and Zelda II on the first Nintendo. I think I can use my video game OCD to my advantage in rehab. It makes total sense to me. I wish I thought of this earlier. Video games are bad for you? I'm just the dork to come up with an "experiment" and test that theory.

Friday, February 22, 2008

Something is not right with this. It seems like 1/2 the young survivors I meet online get really sick or have passed. I've been a "survivor"/"mAss Kicker" for 2 1/2 years now. I find this very disturbing because over the past 30 years there has been no improvement in the survival rates in young adult age group (15-39) while the survival rates in the pediatric and geriatric population have improved. But more importantly this is disturbing to me because this group of young adult patients were the people who I preferred to turn to when I needed support. My friends were there, but it is nice to talk to or email someone that understands what you are up against. For me, most of the brain tumor patients that I could find were older women my mom's age. Now don't get me wrong, hanging out with other survivors was great, but finding young people closer to my age that could speak my "language" was something that I missed. My friends and family were great, but it was so nice to meet someone like me that was walking or had walked a similar path.

There are many reasons there has been no improvement in young adult survival rates:

**\* Lack of research - Young people often are not eligible for studies (too old for pediatric studies or too young for traditional studies) and there are few studies geared towards the 15-39 age group.**
**\* Entry-level jobs with poor healthcare - Young people are just starting out so the costs of healthcare are not a priority. Education about warning signs could really help.**
**\* Doctors don't take us seriously because we are not in the typical demographic for cancer, brain tumors, or whatever**
**\* "Superman" complex - Belief that nothing can happen to us until it's too late. We think we are invincible!**

I'm tired of learning about people I've met getting sick again. I have made many friends on MySpace and facebook, but the fact remains that this demographic is often ignored. Organizations like *I'm Too Young for This* or *Planet Cancer* do a great job providing support for the neglected young adult demographic, but people need to be aware of this fact. Because people generally don't know about this, please spread the word.

Monday, February 25, 2008

I'm starting to get excited! On Thursday, I get to go to Hollywood for a charity comedy night. I'm really excited to meet other young brain tumor survivors. As I mentioned in the previous post, we are hard to find, plus it seems like a lot of the people I meet get sick again. That scares the hell out of me; I'll be looking over my shoulder for the rest of my life. I think I like my odds, but you never know. It will be nice to get away for a little while. I've got a lot of stuff coming up, so this will be like a mini-vacation.

Tuesday, February 26, 2008

I love to eat. Last night I went out with my friends for some sushi. I love going with them for Korean, Japanese, Chinese, Indian, Thai, and Malaysian food because we always eat family style. This means we split all our dishes and the bill equally, which ultimately means more variety for everyone. This is the reason why I love buffets, but that is another story.

Anyways, there is something special about "breaking bread" with people. It's a very intimate gesture. You need to eat to sustain life, so when someone invites me to eat with them I rarely decline. Having a meal with someone means, "You are important enough to sustain my life with." OK, maybe that is a little extreme, but think about it… business meetings take place over lunch, dates revolve around dinner, and breakfast has the reputation of being the most important meal of the day (who was the last person you actually sat down and had breakfast with… I'll bet it was with someone special).

I still eat junk food and stuff that is not good for you. Some people are really strict about their diets for different reasons. I am not one of those people. It is only a matter of time before I need to change my diet. I'm reading more about how your diet can affect your healing and prevent certain impairments. I will still be eating my "Seoul food" with my friends. To me… sharing food with my friends is really my "soul food."

Thursday, March 6, 2008

I spent my entire adult life preparing for a career to help others rehabilitate from catastrophic diagnoses. After almost 2 years working as a physical therapist, I received shocking news that I was the recipient of a catastrophic diagnosis. In September 2005, I was diagnosed with a meningioma, a brain tumor. I became someone I've spent years preparing to help. My eyes have been opened to a world of challenges a brain tumor patient and his loved ones must face everyday. Like all brain tumor and brain cancer patients, I was innocently thrust into a very intimidating world I initially knew very little about. Since I have a background as a physical therapist I thought I knew what I would be up against, but there were many challenges I did not expect. I am still facing physical challenges, but my cognition and determination are 100% if not stronger. I've always been a pretty stubborn guy and I've always liked to do things on my own. When I got home from the hospital everyone wanted to wait on me hand and foot! While most people would indulge in this, I quickly got annoyed by it. I found it very demeaning. I eventually learned to politely decline assistance, but early in my recovery this would infuriate me. One of the toughest things I have to deal with is the fact that I know what I need to do to progress, but I still can't do some of those things quite yet. I'm getting a very REAL lesson on perseverance. The most eye-opening challenge that I have to deal with is the feeling of isolation. I have many friends easily accessible via email/facebook/myspace/instant messaging/phone calls, but I do not know very many people that truly understand the struggles of a brain tumor survivor that have undergone similar experiences. As a young guy, most of the survivors I have met were women my mother's age. I have enjoyed meeting them, but there is only so much you can talk with them about.

My search for other young survivors similar to me led me to Ken Baker and *Head to Hollywood*. I was really excited to finally find someone similar to me that understood what I was dealing with! Ken mentioned that he was one of the directors of *Head to Hollywood* and he would like to invite me to come up to Hollywood for their inaugural comedy night. Without hesitation, I agreed. He said that there would be other young survivors there, so I was excited to finally meet guys like me. I'm not alone! My first dilemma was: who do I take as my complimentary guest? I decided to take my mom because she has been the most popular recipient of my "witty" attitude and she would enjoy the "Hollywood experience" the most out of all my loved ones. She deserved it. My second dilemma was: how am I going to get up there? There is no way I would want my mother driving in L.A. traffic. We could take the train to L.A. from San Diego. My third dilemma was: where are we going to stay in L.A.? *Head to Hollywood* set us up in a fancy hotel room right next to the comedy club on the famous Sunset Strip in Hollywood with a nice view of Sunset Boulevard. Before the event I finally got to meet some young brain tumor survivors face-to-face. We hit it off right away. Again, I was the youngest one there, but at least we were in the same decade! Most of my online buddies I have yet to meet face-to-face. The polite, "choir boy Eric" went into hiding and the mischievous "Naughty Galvez" came out to play! Two of my new brain tumor buddies helped me walk into the venue without the walker. I told them that I had only done this once in public, but I'd like to try it again. Those guys stepped up without asking any questions... pretty cool. It was like having big brothers looking out for you. Later that night they helped me walk all the way back to the hotel room without the walker! I can't believe I had only known them 5 minutes! It was such a small gesture, but it meant the world to me.

On the red carpet we were addressing questions for an interview, but I felt very comfortable around these guys and felt like I had known them for quite some time. It made me smile seeing people wear the "Tumors Suck!" stickers I brought to the event. I thought the comedy show was great! Chelsea Handler and friends were hilarious! They did make quite a few awkward situations for me though. I was stuck sitting between my mom and my friend's dad so I transformed back into "choir boy Eric." Let's say there were a few jokes that evening that weren't of the family variety. I had to sip my Coke and try not to laugh too loud during those awkward situations. I'm very glad the lights were dim in the crowd because I was squirming like the bottom two on American Idol before the break. I still had a lot of fun, though. The evening was packed full of memories that will last a lifetime. *Head to Hollywood* definitely provided me with an escape from the grind and helped me find exactly what I was looking for. I am still continuing to make physical improvements and am excited to see where my next stop in life takes me.

Monday, March 10, 2008

How come no one ever talks about Healthy People 2010? I remembered this from a class in Physical Therapy School. It sounded like a good program then in 2003. Was it just a media fad? Was it just something our professors preached to us in an "ideal world?" I think this is ideally the direction of American healthcare. I really think the physical therapist will play a large role in accomplishing this plan due to our frequent contact with our patients.

Sunday, March 16, 2008

It's that time of year for me to start doing some crazy stuff. Last year I walked the Carlsbad 5000. It took me almost three frickin' hours to do the 3.1 mile race. Looking back, I probably wasn't ready. I was lucky to have my friends there to help me out. I plan on doing it again this year only it will be different. I still need a little help but I intend to walk much faster and I have a purpose this year. I did it last year because selfishly I wanted to finish the race that got me hooked on an active lifestyle. This year is different. Don't get me wrong... I'm still going to crush my time from last year, but it just so happens that April 6-12 is Young Adult Cancer Awareness Week. I will be walking for all my young adult survivor colleagues to raise awareness for this neglected demographic. I got some more crazy stuff planned... stay tuned!

Monday, March 17, 2008

I just found out another one of my online buddies passed away from her battle with a brain tumor. This is very real. This one hurts a little more because she was one of my first online buddies and she was one of the few people who would talk smack with me. I'd give her a hard time about sitting around with her thumb up her butt... and smelling it, while she would call me an overachieving geek/dork/nerd. She had so much attitude, which is probably why we got along so well. She was given a year to live, but we never talked about that. I felt "normal" whenever we talked smack to each other. I can only hope she felt the same way. I knew this was coming, but it still hurts. I'm not good at being sad. I get mad. When I get mad, things happen.

Monday, March 24, 2008

Wow, time has been flying. I'm trying to use my left hand more. Good news is I completed my first song on *Guitar Hero 3*. Only took me a month but it was fun. *Slow Ride...* check. Next up *Talk Dirty to Me*. I'm building up my endurance for Carlsbad. Only 2 more weeks... I will be ready. Damn, I can't wait to start running again. It's getting soooo nice out. As I mentioned earlier April 6-12 is *Young Adult Cancer Awareness Week*. This movement is growing... 'bout time people are taking notice. There are issues like fertility, career, or relationship issues that the pediatric or geriatric population don't have to deal with.

Tuesday, April 1, 2008

Yo Tumor! You're gone but not forgotten! Although I "dumped" you in 2005, I'm still trying to put the pieces back together. Let me tell you again, you picked the wrong guy to mess with. I'm getting stronger everyday and I'm doing things I never dreamed I would do. This is just taking forever! Many new doors are opening for me, but my eyes are still focused on recovering and battling you! I have a few new projects I will unveil in the coming weeks. On Sunday, I'll be walking the Carlsbad

5000 again. Last year I did it for myself. This year I'm doing it for all the young adult survivors! On that note… "F" you Tumor! "luv" Galvez

Tuesday, April 8, 2008

The Carlsbad 5000 went well. Still took me 2 hours, but shaved off 45 minutes from last year… huge improvement! I knew things were going to go well right off the bat because this year I actually put some planning into the preparation and we knew what to expect. I think it helped that I had a purpose this year. Last year I walked because I am stubborn and wanted to prove to myself that it could still be done. This year, I did it to honor all my friends I have met online that are dealing with crap like: cancer, brain tumors, radiation, chemo, recovery from the aforementioned treatments, or waiting for an appropriate time for treatment to commence.

The Carlsbad 5000 is one of the premiere 5K races in the world. 16 world records have been broken there, so it draws thousands of participants each year. Because of that, they hold a number of races for different categories. Three years ago I earned my first medal there. I was very proud of myself because they only give medals to the top 250 in each race! I was hooked and will forever feel a special bond with the Carlsbad. Last year I just wanted to return and finish it. Time was not an issue. This year I wanted to do it for my friends. My first goal this year was to cross the course before the fast runners hit the home stretch. Since the course was a loop, the runners have to cross the start of the race to enter to home stretch. Last year, we had to wait for the fast runners in the first race to pass by at the beginning of our crazy walk before we were allowed to continue my stubborn march. This year we breezed pass the home stretch undetected. Last year we walked through 3 races (got passed and smoked by everyone… a very humbling experience). This year I got to cross the finish line with the "stragglers" in my age group. Even though I had a one and half hour head start two races prior it felt so good finishing with guys my age. For a little while, I felt like I was where I belonged.

One of my biggest problems throughout my rehab (and before brain surgery) is that I am easily distracted. I'm really glad I had my friends there whispering in my ear to stay focused. So many people were shouting words of encouragement. How do you ignore that? I always want to acknowledge people, but it would always throw me off. Once I'm focused on a task, good things usually happen, but when I lose that focus that when things break down. I'm getting better though! Anyways, I didn't look up at all in the home stretch. There were a lot of people there, but the funny thing is I didn't see any of them.

There were a few cameras waiting for us at the finish line, which was pretty cool. We got to spread a little awareness. This week is National Young Adult Cancer Awareness Week. Tumors Suck stickers are being passed out all over the US and Canada! They will be available to everyone real soon!

We are planning a "field trip" to SeaWorld in San Diego on Saturday to end *National Young Adult Cancer Awareness Week*. Some more stuff is in the works the next few months, but getting ready to catch some waves this summer is a high priority…

Saturday, April 12, 2008

I spent the entire day outside in sunny 80 degree San Diego weather at Sea World! You can hate me, if you live somewhere cold and rainy. I'm 32 years old but I love that place! I'm in San Diego damn it! So I sure as hell am going to enjoy myself and take advantage of my time here! I think it is amazing to see intelligent creatures, like orcas (killer whales) and dolphins, perform coordinated tricks. I always feel like a little kid whenever I go there. I can't contain my "ooohs" and "aaahs." My inner nerd is always satisfied by the little tidbits of info I pick up. (Did you know flamingos are pink because of the high content of shrimp they eat? I question the validity of this statement because shrimp don't turn pink till you cook them.) Anyways, I've got a year pass, so by the end of the year I want to try walking the park. My ulterior motive in going today was to scope out the bench locations. I'm happy to see that there are many places to sit in the park, but my concerns are distractions and crowds. I am already thinking of trying this in the fall or early winter when there are no tourists.

I have already set my sights on returning to the beach this summer. I do need to take care of a few things first. This weekend I am attending my first brain tumor conference at UCLA. Then on Sunday I will be a guest on *Vital Options-The Group Room*. It is an international radio show distributed on XM Radio. I'll be a panelist discussing unique issues with minority survivors. Tune in if you can; there will be some interesting perspectives. It will be broadcast online and in select markets. Please check the website for details. On May 9, I am 1 of 4 recipients of the *Sharp Eagle Spirit Award*. I just learned this is a $150/plate event! Ooooo fancy smancy!

Tuesday, April 22, 2008

This weekend was packed full of excitement! On Thursday afternoon I took the train up to L.A. again because I really wanted to attend a free brain tumor conference at UCLA. I went by myself hoping to find some additional insight into to my condition and see if the experts there had any new advice for me. It was great to see some familiar faces there, and make some new friends. I brought some "TUMORS SUCK" stickers with me, and by the end of the conference everyone was wearing one! They were a big hit! I found the conference very enlightening; however I did not find the new advice from the experts I was looking for. Since my case is so unique, and it is relatively early, I will just have to be content waiting and continue to do what I am doing. I am still progressing, but I want to do everything in my power to nurture this process.

Friday was the first day of the conference. I now realize that, based on the location of my tumor between the brain stem and cerebellum, I am either really brave or really stubborn/dumb. Actually, I think I can lean towards the stubborn/dumb side. To take that kind of a risk you really have to be a little of both, but you have to be fully aware of the consequences. I consider myself VERY lucky, so I am not taking

ANYTHING for granted! I'm not out of the water yet, but I feel like I am back in control (to a certain extent). I had the opportunity to pick some of the smartest brains in neuro-oncology and I still haven't heard any new advice on how to handle the ataxia in my left arm and the intention tremor in my right arm other than "keep doing what you are doing." My expertise is rehabilitation, but no doctor knows exactly what to do with me next. I am convinced that if I sit around and wait, things will not progress for me. I will have to take things into my own hands. Friday night, I got to meet up with some friends in Santa Monica. We have laid the groundwork for some fun activities this summer. Oooooo... It's gonna be so fun!

Saturday was day two of the conference. It was definitely more intimate than the first day with breakout sessions, so there was more room to ask questions. I think I enjoyed the conference more the second day. Looking around the rooms I noticed that I really stuck out. Not only was I one of the youngest guys in the room, but also walking slowly with the walker draws a lot of unwanted attention. I'm glad I've learned to ignore it. I realize that right now I still need the walker to walk with "modified independence." The dilemma I face now is whether to practice with the cane or no assistive device. The cane throws things off when I'm walking because the tremors in my right arm make cane placement unsteady. The ataxia in my left arm makes holding the cane stable very difficult. I am trying to problem solve this dilemma, so for now the walker has to do. The thing is, the walker is so bulky... try a quad cane? I am fine walking with someone holding my elbow, but I'm not independent. Saturday night, I was exhausted after a long day. Me and my buddy grabbed some sushi and hung out at a friend's place to play a little *Guitar Hero 3*. I was in bed by midnight! Whoa... in bed on a Saturday night by 12 on a trip to L.A.!

Sunday, was my radio debut on the *Vital Options Group Room* on XM Radio. I still speak a little slower than normal, but Selma, the host, did a great job getting everyone involved. I'll post a link to it once it is available online. Being a part of the show was a great experience. I was expecting to go to a small back room. Turns out it was in one of the largest radio studios in L.A., premier radio network. Someone told me Jim Rome, the sports show host, does his show there! For a second I thought, "For a normally quiet guy, what are you getting yourself into?" Everything I'm doing is very uncharacteristic for me. There were two other young adult survivors in the studio and 3 other guests called in, so my nervousness quickly resolved. I really enjoyed meeting the other young survivors. It was the first time I had participated in a "support group" type session. Figures I had to go all out for my first session. Anyways, the show went well and was actually quite fun for everyone involved. I'm looking forward to doing it again. Sunday night I got to meet up with some friends I hadn't seen in a long time. A lot has happened in the past 2 years, but it was great to see that people are still the same.

I had to catch a late night bus to San Diego. I totally went old school traveling to L.A. on a train/bus. It was kind of neat sitting in Union Station knowing that this was the primary means of transportation before commercial airlines, greenhouse gases, or air pollution. It was a simpler time then. Not to mention, this form of travel is much "greener" than driving a car up there. I didn't get the answers I was looking for in L.A., but the contacts I made and have re-established made my throwback travel well worth the effort.

Monday, May 5, 2008

Physically I'm still making progress returning to what I would normally be doing. This is taking a REALLY long time. I consider myself to be a very lucky man, but in order to keep my sanity and appease the creative beast within me, I've had to resort to a kinder gentler time... my childhood. Ah yes, those were the days of eating sugary cereal, coloring, writing in notebooks, playing video games, etc. Well, I've taken the "developmental" theories/progressions and applied them to my own rehab. Why not have fun with it, right?

I'm trying to use my left hand more everyday so I try to eat a bowl of cereal as a lefty (I still like fruit loops… sue me), I have an old Anatomy coloring book from school I never used so I'm coloring as a lefty, and writing with my left hand is like starting from scratch. Just holding a pen in the proper position is huge adjustment. Don't think it's all work and no play. I just started playing video games again. The Wii has really good potential to be used as a rehab piece of equipment. Core stability/coordination programs could be developed. *Mario Kart* is one of the few games that can get curse words out of me. hahaha! Some more stuff is coming up. I'm meeting some pretty well connected people. This Friday, I get to go to some fancy award banquet.

Monday, May 12, 2008

It seems like I live for the weekends. That hasn't changed since the surgery. That is the only time people are free to do anything lately. This past Friday I was 1 of 4 recipients of the *SHARP Healthcare Victories of Spirit Eagle Award*. The award is given to individuals who overcome the odds and give back to the community. All of the recipients are former rehab patients who have more than exceeded their recovery. Getting this award came as a total surprise to me because I am still in the heat of my own recovery. Just seeing what the other recipients had to endure and how far they've come along gives me a lot of hope. I'm getting a very real lesson in patience.

Both my parents were present for the ceremony as well as many of my friends, colleagues, and former co-workers. I had a smile on my face the whole night. I'm told there were 575 guests at the semi-formal event: corporate sponsors, physicians, clinicians, the board of directors… thank God I didn't have to say anything! They showed very powerful videos highlighting each recipient's journey. There wasn't a dry eye in the room at the end of the night. Many more doors are opening up for me.

Later that evening I met up with some friends at a bar downtown. More my element. I could not put up with wearing a suit or even a tie everyday. I feel like it has been a long time since I've been downtown. I realize now how much I miss live music. Was cool just hanging out. I've talked about returning to driving in the past, it's time to seriously start prepping for it. I've just learned how to play *Mario Kart* online... hee hee... oh boy! Everyone tells me once you can drive again, you reach another "level" in rehab.

Thursday, May 22, 2008

Well, I'm back in Michigan for the next two weeks. Some crazy stuff is starting to happen. I'm leaving just when things are starting to get interesting. I just got a Mac and I've been playing around with iMovie. Check out some of my old videos on my blog. More on the way.

My fall schedule is really getting full. I'm a confirmed speaker in Boston, Ann Arbor, and Philly! Scary thing is I've got more stuff in the works. Funniest thing was I found an old journal I was keeping from 1995 on my trip to the Philippines and California for a convention. The journal is 12 years old! Weird reading my thoughts as a 20-year-old. I am in the process of adding to the journal as a lefty. So far my entries have only been the alphabet, but as soon as my writing improves I'll make real entries as a lefty.

Last weekend was pretty laid back. Family came to visit, so we did the touristy stuff. I'm still in awe of this place, San Diego, I call home!

Thursday, May 29, 2008

It's so nice being back in Michigan. I'm here for another week. I came back because I was a groomsman in my old roommate's wedding. I've had the honor of standing in three weddings since my surgery in 2005. In the first one, I needed a wheelchair to go up the aisle at the end of the ceremony. In the second one, I used a walker. In this one, I walked up the aisle holding onto my partner and had a friend close by in case I stumbled. Well, I made it without falling. I keep making progress, but I am not even close to being satisfied yet. This summer is time to hit the beach for "surfing" again. I think a more realistic goal is paddling out to the line-up and sitting on my board.

I got a few more things up my sleeve. Many doors are opening to keep me busy. I'm meeting a lot of new friends. I'm enjoying everything.

Saturday, June 14, 2008

Things definitely aren't boring. I always seem to find ways to keep myself busy. I just restarted physical therapy. I think I am at the point where I can't progress any further on my own. I need help now. I'm now receiving therapy where I was working when I got thrown a curve ball. Everyone was there when I found out. I have different therapists than when I was in the hospital, but they are still my colleagues. I am on the other side again. I still wish to return to the profession I love, but I am starting to realize that I may have a larger calling. I still plan on hitting the beach this summer. My eyes are set on getting on a surfboard again.

Monday, June 16, 2008

*Summer summer summertime. Time to sit back and unwind.* Words from Will Smith's (AKA *the Fresh Prince* in another life) classic hit *Summertime.* This summer, I'm returning to the basics. I'm going to focus on rehab and writing. No more doing all this promotion/advocacy stuff. I need a break. It is hard work! I can see how people can throw themselves into it. When you have a passion for a cause it is easy to motivate yourself to work for that cause. I've never been behind a computer screen so long! I want to try to thank everyone that supported me. I just got a Mac so I'm screwing around on it. I'm going to hit the beach soon. Can't wait to battle the waves again.

Saturday, June 21, 2008

Walked down to the pool yesterday, holding onto the boogie board without the cane. First time I've done that. Getting down there was not a problem. It felt really good going down there holding the board. I feel so much closer to normalcy. I slapped on some sunscreen and did a couple laps around the pool. A couple years ago I would have been really self-conscious about having so many gawkers but now… I don't care. I can tell there is improvement. People who haven't seen me for a while always tell me there is improvement. I appreciate all the complements on my progress, and I love to hear them, but I am not satisfied. When I stop hearing those complements than it means a plateau in progress has been reached. There will always be room for improvement. I restarted official therapy because I have new insurance. I think it is justified because the first time around therapy was focused on "adapting" to my physical impairments because nobody knew what to do with me. This time around I want to "rehabilitate" the physical impairments. Nobody knows still what to do with me, but I have a better idea of what I am capable of doing.

I start official aquatic PT next week so I made up some of my own exercises with the boogie board. Hahaha! After my warm up lap, I did the few aquatic exercises I knew, then paddled a few more laps on the boogie board surfboard style. After the kids in the pool left I had the water all to myself. Aahhh… I laid in the water with my head tilted back and hair in the cool water. The board under my arms kept me afloat on my back as my toes floated towards the surface on the other side of the board. The sun kept my face warm while my body was cool in the water. I shut my eyes. When I opened them again, I squinted and saw three palm trees and a clear blue sky. *I'm alive.* I shut my eyes again for a little while. My feet hit something. I must have drifted into the wall. I scrambled to get away from the wall. Oops. This is the deeper end. Was not expecting that. I can hold my breath a long time. Freaked out a few sunbathers and my pops. They rush to my aid! Hello Reality. Cause a little commotion. I assure them I'm OK. No problem, just under water… jeez. I've never been the kind of guy to just get up and go. I need a little buffer before I start going after a nap. I can't take power naps because if I'm out, it will take me a while to start going again. In the morning, I have to wake up early to get alert before I can function. That embarrassing incident ended my afternoon at the pool.

Sunday, I test out my new surfboard. Just got it. I also got a life jacket cause I think this summer I might be trying some things a little more "challenging." : )

Saturday, June 23, 2008
A PHYSICAL THERAPY S.O.A.P. NOTE ON ME BY ME(THE PHYSICAL THERAPIST)

S: "I'm excited to test this thing out, but dude it's early"

O: 9AM, 6/22/08, La Jolla Shores. 80 and sunny. Clear sky. 1-3' calm waves. Water temp 67 degrees.

A: Beach was crowded. Parking difficult on beautiful day. I immediately wanted to try paddling out to the line up. The line-up is where all the surfers sit and wait on their boards for a good wave to ride. This was one of my favorite parts of surfing. Here, I would hang out with my friends in the morning to watch the horizon and just chill, which usually meant making fun of each other. You really felt humbled out there looking at the vastness of the ocean, the sounds of the water, the refreshing breeze on your face, the brisk smell of the salt water. Ahhhh. I used to love going out there before work with a couple of my coworkers just to unwind. I now understand why surfers are so laid back. Don't get me wrong, I get excited to catch a good wave. I am by no means a "Zen master," but I do appreciate that state of mind.

The first few times out on the new board were trial and error. The first time out, my assistants launched me on the first big wave that hit the line up. I was like "Wait! We just got heeeere!" I wanted to soak in returning to the line up. The new board is shorter than the previous boards I've practiced on so I had to find a new standing balance point. I did make it out to the line-up again and sat on the board for about 3 minutes. I only fell off once cause I got cocky and tried wiping my nose.

I could have done this all morning, but I figured my assistants needed a break. They were treading water beside me the whole time! You can't be a slouch if you want to help me out! I'll push you!

I went back to the white wash to try standing and figure out the board. The white wash is easier to catch waves in because they are more frequent and a little more "predictable." I found out where the balance point is on the board. I figured out that I'm pushing too heavily with my right arm causing the board to tilt when I pop up. I need to take into account the speed of the board on the wave. I also need to take into account the slipperiness of the board.

P: Continue home pop-up simulations on the boogie board. Mark board for balance point. Arrive earlier so the beach is less crowded. Sitting balance core stability training. More Swiss ball - rotation activities? Turning surf board in sitting. Sitting to prone on board. Climbing on board to prone independently. Re-assess standing goal in white wash at onset of next "session."

Eric Galvez PT DPT CSCS

Wednesday, July 2, 2008

Yesterday I used the stair master for the first time in months. I have really lost my lungs. I was only able to get 7 minutes at Level 5. Weak sauce. Guess what I'll be working on… I'm also noticing that I really don't get out much… been so busy lately. The only time I see people are when they come to visit me. It's been a really long time since I've been able to see anyone by myself. I have to depend on other people for rides. I am a freshman in high school again! That is going to have to change. I'm forcing myself to fold up that walker now.

This book could go on forever, but I choose to end my story here. All of our lives will go on. My story isn't even close to being finished! I am playing with house money right now so I'm taking a lot of risks I normally wouldn't be taking. I have done pretty well so far. Hey, you're reading this sentence right now. I never dreamed I would pull this book off. It all started with a simple phrase… "Why not?" I didn't have a good answer so voila… a book! It goes to show you that the ONLY THING LIMITING YOURSELF… IS YOURSELF! Failure doesn't scare me as much as it used to. I will always pick myself up and brush the dirt off my shoulders when I fall. I'm not perfect and I do fall a lot, but I'll get up every time! I've got more stuff up my sleeve. I invite you to check out my blog www.ericgalvezdpt.com to see what else is going on or to see what is going on with me now. I really think this book is just the beginning. I will try to update the blog periodically, but we'll see how long that lasts. Stay tuned! Drop me a line!

# Photograph

Every memory of walking out the front door
I found the photo of the friend that I was looking for
It's hard to say it, time to say it
Goodbye, goodbye.

**-Nickelback,** *All the Right Reasons* 2005

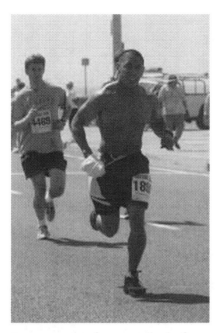

Figure 1. At a race a few months before surgery

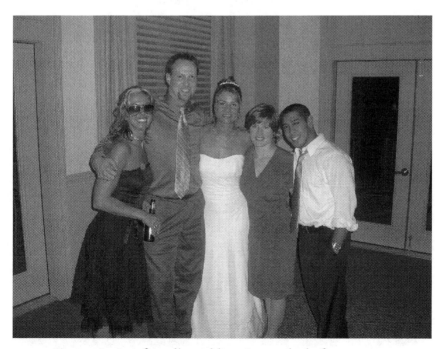

Figure 2. At a friend's wedding 2 months before surgery

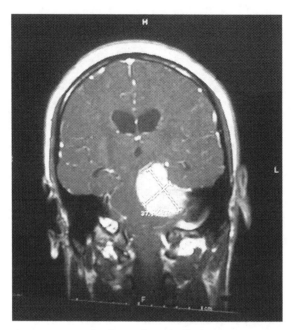

Figure 3. Can you see the big white ball that's not supposed to be there? It's not in the greatest spot!

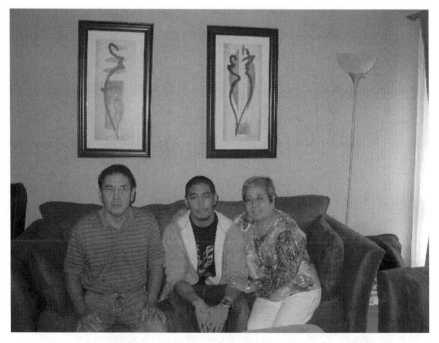

Figure 4. With my Mom and Dad the day before surgery.

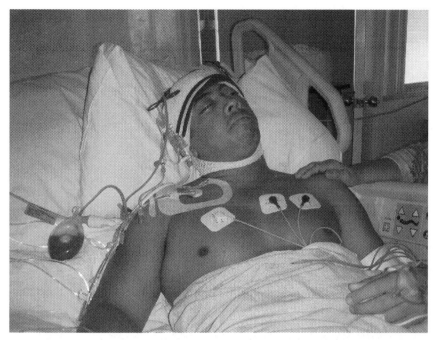

Figure 5. In ICU with my post-surgical headgear and tubes.

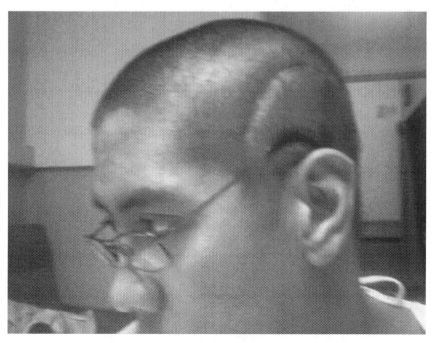

Figure 6. My cool new scar.

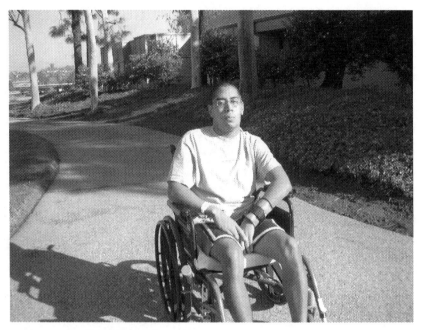

Figure 7. Catching some rays. I lost some weight, but I got it back thanks to the cookies everyone gave me.

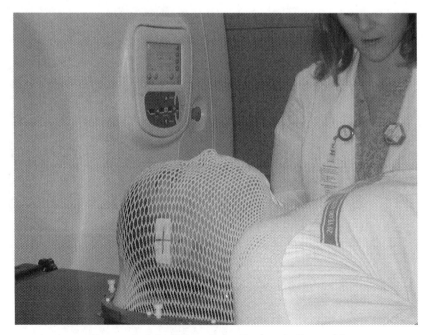

Figure 8. My "Han Solo Carbonite" mask!

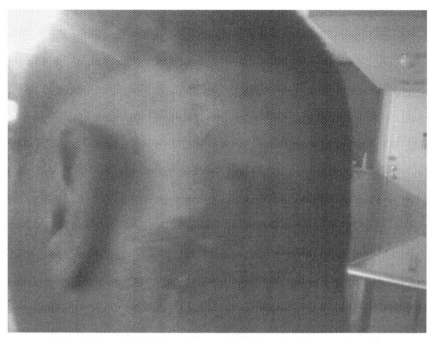

Figure 9. The effects of radiation therapy.

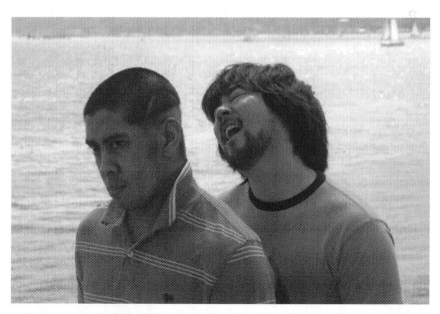

Figure 10. My friend Gene goofs off while a look of determination
forms on my face

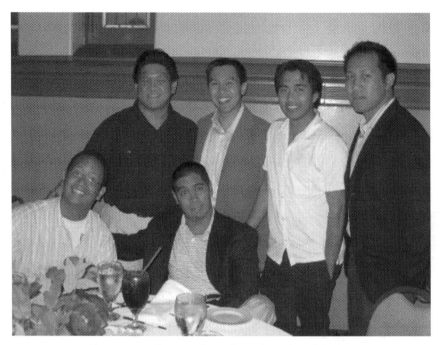

Figure 11. Some of my friends in Michigan.

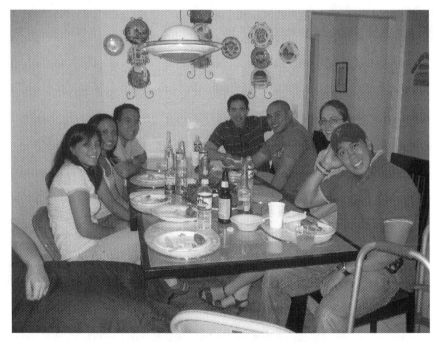

Figure 12. My Michigan family.

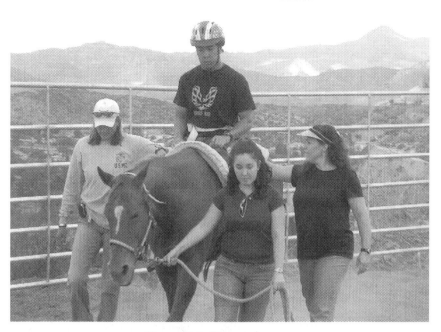

Figure 13. Hippotherapy

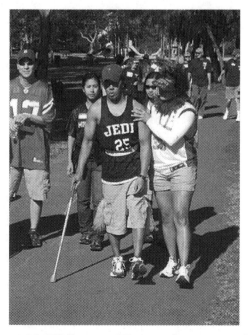

Figure 14. Walking a 5K, one of my crazy ideas

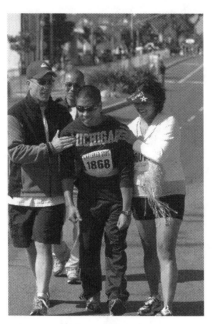

Figure 15. Walking the Carsbad 5000,
I could not have done it without Machi, Dan, and Oliver

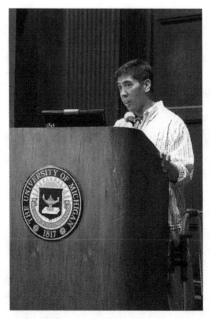

Figure 16. People are actually listening to me at the
University of Michigan book signing!

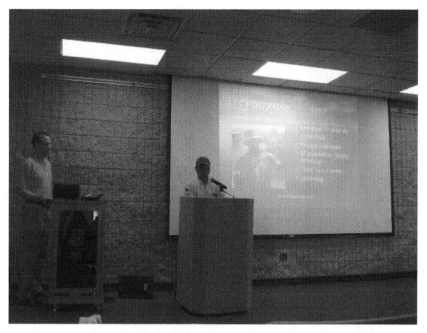

Figure 17. I'm getting more used to public speaking.
Still don't like it though!

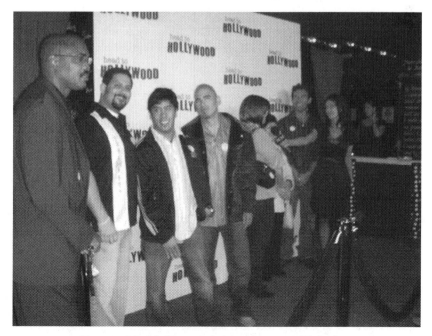

Figure 18. Hollywood, here I come! Hahaha!

# Part II:
# Perspectives

# Stand By Me

If the sky that we look upon
Should tumble and fall
And the mountains should crumble to the sea
I won't cry, I won't cry, no I won't shed a tear
Just as long as you stand, stand by me

**-Ben E King**, *single* 1961

I am who I am because of my family. I got my obsessive compulsiveness, tenacity, and ability to love from my mom. I got my impatience, work ethic, and charm from my dad. I developed my sense of humor and laid back demeanor with my brother. When all of us are together there is a good balance. Family is very important in the Filipino culture. Loyalty to your parents is very highly regarded. A lot of times the kids in a close family don't leave the house until they are married. I'm surprised my parents didn't have very many objections when I told them I was moving to California. I was the model son growing up and always listened to my parents. I was the "good" kid who got good grades and stayed out of trouble at school, and my brother was the rebel who got caught drinking and smoking. As we got older, our roles slightly reversed. I moved away from home and wanted to start my own life while my brother stayed close to home, bought my mom a puppy, and played in a golf league with my dad. I also became a sarcastic smart-ass towards both my parents when I started my rehab.

My mom is a very typical overprotective Filipina mom. She talks a lot. She has to have her hand in everything and sweats over small insignificant details. She puts me and my brother ahead of everyone else. According to her, we are the best looking and most eligible bachelors on the face of the Earth. She also has a knack for handing out advice to us on things she knows very little or nothing about. This really got on my nerves when she would try to give me PT advice. Whenever she told me to do anything, I either ignored her or asked her, "Why? What muscles are involved? Do you remember what I do for a living?" She tried to be helpful, but in the end she always succeeded in pissing me off because I wanted to do everything on my own. I know I was a little pigheaded whenever I tried to be independent. I got really mad whenever I felt like I was being coddled. How she put up with 3 boys: me, my brother, and my dad. I have no idea! She deserves a medal or something.

Around Christmas, when I first got home from rehab, I was washing my face at the sink with a face towel. My mom was lecturing me at the time about how I should scrub my face. Of course, I was ignoring her. She grabbed the face towel out of my hand and started washing my face for me! I was so mad! Just like a little kid, I tried to get away. I was still in the wheelchair at the time, so I tried to wheel away. I didn't succeed. She actually chased me down in the wheelchair and finished scrubbing my face for me. I've never seen her move so fast! That hasn't happened since I was 7 years old! I was so pissed off! I just sat there and pouted while she finished scrubbing my face! How humiliating! Thank God no one was around! I can now laugh at the picture of her chasing me down in the wheelchair trying to scrub my face. She's gotten better as the months passed, but I still catch her staring at me with "mother eyes." She used to bring up stuff from when I was a toddler, like lying down on the floor to put on my jacket or how hard it was for me learning to tie my shoes. In her eyes I was that little kid again. I jokingly told my brother to get some random girl pregnant just to get her off my back. Given everything I've been through I can now laugh at everything, but at the time it really pissed me off. I made her watch Disney and Pixar's *Finding Nemo* to drive home the idea that although I'm not 100% yet, there is still a lot I can do on my own if given a chance.

My dad is a very pessimistic man. He doesn't like high expectations, which eventually lead to disappointment. Growing up, my brother and I were terrified of his belt and slipper. Just a slow count to 3 from him would straighten out any mischievous activities we were doing or thinking about doing. At the end of the 3 count he would grab us by the ear, drag us to him, and spank our mischievous little butts. While we were scared of him, we always knew he was looking out for us. One night when I was little, I told him that the neighborhood bully was giving us a hard time on our walk home from school. He told me not to worry and to just keep walking. The following day the bully wasn't around. Lucky for him. I caught a glimpse of my dad's car tailing us like an undercover policeman as we were walking home. He was trying to hide, but I saw him. I shudder to think of what would have ensued if that bully gave us a hard time that afternoon.

My dad is a lot more laid back than my Mom, so I was OK with him staying with me in San Diego. Lucky for me he had just retired so he was able to come out San Diego to stay with me before the surgery and while I recovered.

He was diagnosed with Parkinsons-like symptoms in 2002. He has a slight hand tremor and a little rigidity. Everything is well controlled with medication, but I have a hard time accepting the fact that it is Parkinsons Disease. At first it was a little weird watching the man I admired growing up get weaker before my eyes. At that point, I realized that everyone gets old. Nothing lasts forever. Don't dwell on the past because the future isn't written yet, so just enjoy the now.

My dad needed to know what was going on all the time. I started to walk with him in the hallways at my apartment. Every time I would stumble, he would ask, "What happened there?" When he first started doing it, I would give him a long and drawn-out technical PT answer. He always nodded as if he understood what I was saying. After a while his questions got annoying so my replies would get shorter and more vague. "What happened there?" My new response would be, "I fell." Then I would start walking again. He always put up a very pessimistic attitude when ever I wanted to try something new. The last thing I wanted or needed to hear from anyone was a negative attitude. This was how he always was, so I just ignored it. I think he was more scared of me falling then I was. He always wanted me to take the safest and slower route. My brother, on the other hand, didn't care and would still challenge me.

My brother, Oliver, and I were very competitive growing up. We still are competitive. When I told him about the tumor he just said, "You're too tough. Just beat it." Not a hint of fear in him. It was exactly what I needed to hear. Everyone else I told about the tumor would get really emotional and break down in front of me. Of course, seeing people upset made me upset. I guess you should cry to let things out. I tried crying on my own, but it just wasn't working. Every time I tried, I would end up sounding like a broken lawn mower. Picture a grown man taking deep breaths and trying to let "sad" sounds leave his mouth. I ended up just laughing at my pathetic self. The only time I could cry was if someone was crying with me. I couldn't do it alone. The mere thought of Oliver's confidence helped me believe that I was gonna be OK. The whole time I was going through rehab, I never felt sorry for myself. I would rather just focus on getting better.

My cousins came out to visit me, as well, after the surgery. My cousin Alvin came out first while I was in the hospital; Aileen and her husband Jason came to San Diego when I first got home; Tina, Gilbert and his wife Becky came to visit after I was at home for a few months. I got to see some of my other cousins and family in June at a family reunion. These cousins were much younger, still in high school or college. I would let them sit in the wheelchair while I pushed them around. I let them experiment with it: propelling it, maneuvering in the bathroom, or going to dinner in it. I wanted them to know what I was going through. I hope it made them realize how difficult it is living with a physical impairment.

I missed Aileen and Jason's wedding because I was going through pre-op preparations and I was unable to travel. All my cousins were there. It was the first of many events I would miss, so it was really great that they came out to see me. When the last set of cousins came to visit, I promised myself that I wouldn't miss another major event. I was still scheduled to be the best man at one of my best friend's wedding.

Many of my co-workers came to visit me in the hospital. When I first started working, I worked as an acute therapist on the orthopedic floor. I saw many total knee, total hip patients, back/neck surgery patients, and ironically a few craniotomy patients. After a few months, I transferred departments when an opening popped up in the satellite outpatient orthopedics clinic. Here I would see patients with neck/back, knee, shoulder, and foot/ankle pain. I still knew many of the acute care and rehab therapists when I had my surgery. It was a little strange at first taking commands from my peers. It took me a while to realize that they were seeing things I couldn't see. I seriously thought this would be a piece of cake and I could treat myself. I eventually realized that my perception of my impairments was incomplete and I should listen to what they were saying. It was time to swallow my pride and do what I need to do to progress. I was really an actual patient now! Actually, it was kind of cool seeing how my co-workers handled each situation. We would share different treatment ideas. I think I asked the different therapists to address my parents more then me so that my parents would understand what was going on. This would be very important because I would tell my parents the exact same thing, but if it came from the mouth of a "real" professional other than me, it carried more weight. I always asked my parents if they had any questions before we ended each session because I'm sure a lot of "shop talk" was involved in my therapy sessions. Things were less strange when I progressed to outpatient therapy because we kept the continuity of care and I stayed with the same therapists. These guys would become my confidants and good friends.

I had many friends come visit me in the hospital and at home. The great thing was I didn't have to ask them to come, they just came. They kept coming and coming. They had to put a sign on my door to limit the amount of visitors I had in my room at one time. It was probably because my friends were too loud and obnoxious for my neighbors to handle. Actually it was probably because a large number of guests were too much of a stimulus and I needed rest. I'm so grateful that I had so many visitors, but I wished I could have spoken more clearly to them. As the months progressed, the number of guests dwindled. Part of it was me not returning calls; the other part was probably their busy lives taking over. This is what I expected. A lot of people were there in the beginning, but only a handful were there at the end. At this point, this handful of people stop becoming your friends, they somehow transform into your family. Don't get me wrong, the people that are first there are great friends, but the people who are tenacious enough to stand by you till the end are the GREATEST friends. Family will always be there to see you through. However annoying they get, they are the ones that will pick you up when you need it.

This has probably been the hardest on my parents. I feel like they were used to seeing me as an athlete. I'm at a very peculiar stage in my life. I still get pimples, but I am also starting to get grey hairs. I'm starting my professional career, but my parents still see me as a 12-year-old child. I get pretty defensive when I feel like I am being "babied." This probably hurt my parents because they just wanted me to get better. My friends and family picked up on this pretty early, but it's probably hard to break the parental instinct.

Many people are affected when a patient goes through rehab. The following pages are the accounts of the people closest to me as I was going through the rehab process. These are the people I interacted with the most during my "rehab sabbatical." Their perspectives are very important because an intimidating diagnosis affects more people than just the patients. It is very important to note his or her perspectives because while a patient is receiving their surgery or treatments, these are the people that stand by helplessly as they watch their son, daughter, father, mother, friend or loved one fight for his or her life. These essays tell their side of the story in my remarkable rehab saga.

# Family Perspectives

# Family Business

*Oliver Galvez*

This is family business
And this is for the family that can't be with us
**-Kanye West**, *The College Dropout* 2004

I don't like having anyone I know in the hospital. It's the feeling of helplessness that really gets to me. I can't do anything, they can't do anything, and it's all up to the doctors. Very cold, businesslike. I am Eric's younger brother. When we were kids, our parents took care of all our bumps and bruises, and I felt more secure knowing that the person "fixing" the problem loved us... As most people with siblings, you have your good times and bad. Growing up we would have our little fights (mostly verbal because he knows I would dominate him!!!), and being guys, we would just shrug them off and act "normal" to each other one hour later. As teenagers we played a lot of the same sports and were very competitive in them and against each other. I still remember the day I beat Eric in the 100-meter dash at the State Championship team meet. I was still a freshman; he was a junior. From that day forward, Eric has yet to beat me in a foot race. In football, Eric was a defensive back and I was a wide receiver so we were matched up a lot in practice. The coaches would play the "are you going to let your brother beat you" game every day. Needless to say, I got the better of Eric on most days. Even with all the sibling rivalries, I won't admit this to his face: I've always looked up to the guy.

Let me give you a brief description about myself. I work for a family-owned retail store in Ann Arbor, Michigan and have been there for almost eight years. I sell custom Audio Distribution Systems and Home Theaters, TV's, Audiophile grade stereos and home entertainment furniture. I also am trying to buy as much property I can afford (or not afford). As of now I own a condo and a duplex. I currently live in the duplex. I try to work out 3-4 days a week running, biking, weight lifting, and various other activities to keep myself in shape. I'm a smoker of more than a decade (I'm quitting when I turn 30). I love my family but I don't express it as much as I should. That's about it I guess.

I remember the day when Eric called and told me about the tumor. At first, I thought that he was messing with me. I couldn't believe that my older brother, who in my eyes was the most physically and mentally tough person I know, was sick!! A few months earlier, I went to see him in San Diego and went to Vegas with him for his 30th birthday. I guess this was when the first signs of the tumor were showing. I knew nothing about this stuff but what was strange was that he seemed normal to me. When I look back at it, he never complained about anything.

Anyways, after a while talking to Eric on the phone, he told me that he thought our mom and dad were taking it pretty hard and asked me to go to their place and hang out with them. I agreed, but a lot of things were going through my head. How could this happen to someone in my family? If it were to happen to anyone it should be me. I draink more than him. I smoke. Why is this happening to my brother!? After I got off the phone with Eric, I just sat in my chair in shock and something happened to me I hate admitting... I cried. I don't know for how long but I can tell you that I really didn't want to believe he was sick. I had to gather myself before I went to my parent's house. I felt that I needed to be strong for my family and most of all for Eric. For some reason I knew that he would be okay. Someone who has the willpower and determination of this guy would defiantly make his come back smooth like Michael Jordan. That is all that has gone though my mind since that day.

I went home to my parents' place to find that they were pretty calm, but I could see in their eyes that they were hiding their worries. I guess it runs in the family. One very fortunate thing that seemed to come at the right time was that my Dad had just retired a few months before all this happened. He was to go to San Diego and care for my brother. I don't remember much else from this night because honestly not much was said except for questions like: *Is it cancer? When is the surgery going to happen? How did it happen? Do you think Eric is alright right now? When are you flying out? How are you guys doing? When does he see the doctor next? Can he come to Michigan for treatment?*

I can't recall when we found out the tumor was non-malignant, but that was a big relief. From that point forward I knew that he was going to be money the rest of the way. The months before the surgery, I made periodic calls to my parents and Eric to see how things were going. I guess he was on some crazy drugs that would make him lose his appetite and feel groggy all the time.

Fast forward to surgery time. With both my parents in San Diego, I was all alone at my parents place. I believe even one of my aunts went there for support, as well. The day of the surgery was a VERY LONG day. I was at work but I couldn't really concentrate on what I was doing. I tried to act normal since I didn't tell anyone this was happening except for my boss, who is also a friend of mine. As the day went on, I would make a call to my mom or dad to see how things were. The most common answer was "I don't know; he is still in surgery." This was starting to freak me out. Eric told me it would take some time but it was nearing half a day!! Throughout the day I would get calls from family and some of Eric's friends telling me if I needed anything they would help out and they wanted to know how the surgery was going. I would just tell them he's still in there and I'm good, Eric is a bad ass. He'll be fine. I was right.

The first time I saw Eric was at Christmas. It was weird. I never thought that I would ever see him in a wheelchair unless it was due to something athletic like snowboarding or until he was 90 years old. That feeling soon passed as we hung out together a little more and then it was just like old times. I would make fun of him and vice versa. He still was the same old Eric but now he sounded like Larry Flynt! (Watch the movie *The People vs. Larry Flynt*…exact same voice I swear to God!) Our mom and dad were very protective but I thought it was understandable. Their eldest son was hurt and all they wanted to do was "fix" him. He gets pissed about it sometimes but I know he loves the fact they still and always will try to make the boo boo's go away.

My first experience with Eric outside of his place was at a family reunion cruise to Alaska. It was good to see that he was improving. His speech was better (no more Larry Flynt). He didn't want to use his wheelchair as much but offshore excursions required it. On the boat, Eric would push me and some cousins around in the wheelchair to practice walking. All he wanted to do was practice walking. I finally told him to get on the treadmill in the gym. The thing I noticed the most about the cruise was that everyone would stare at Eric. People we would walk past or stand in an elevator with would take a long look at my older brother, then at me. He took it all in stride, letting it go and not making a big deal of it. I remember the first dinner we had on the cruise, Eric and I both ordered steak. When we were served, the waiter grabbed the steak knife from Eric's hand and cut his steak for him. I kind of let out a chuckle when I saw this. Eric's expression was priceless. The cruise was definitely eye-opening.

Eric is going to persevere through this. He is a warrior. I hate to see him in this state but I know that when he is fully recovered he will be a better man for it. I have to thank God for the amazing timing of my dad's retirement along with his constant efforts in helping Eric work through this. Our mom is a bit protective of him right now but I'm sure he knows it's only because she loves him. I still look up to Eric even more so now than before. He is and will always be my friend, my nemesis, my teammate, but most of all, my brother.

# High Hopes

*Jose Galvez*

Once there was a silly old ram
Thought he'd punch a hole in a dam
No one could make that ram, scram
He kept buttin' that dam

**-Frank Sinatra**, *The Capitol Years* 1990

A son grows up, moves away, and finds a good job. A father is not supposed to be worried about him anymore. Right? Before I proceed, I would like to thank God for aiding and supporting me and my family through this trying time. It has made me closer to God. I have sought comfort and guidance since the time I learned of Eric's brain tumor. I felt so helpless. I know how dangerous craniotomies are. I have asked people about this kind of tumor. Some are very hopeful; some are more technical referring to the location and size of the mass.

Lots of tests were done to ensure a safe and proper way to go about the operation. Unfortunately, he had a reaction with his angiogram. He called us from the ER a few hours after his angiogram. I rushed to San Diego as soon as possible to keep him company. Medications were prescribed to ease the symptoms caused by the tumor and swelling which made his life a little better. My own medication made it easier for me to handle everything!

I knew he was physically and emotionally affected but he kept a brave front, better than me. I was nervous about the operation, knowing the uncertainty and danger of it. My wife and sister, who is a physician in New York, were here for the surgery. That day was the longest day we experienced. With all the possible scenarios running through our minds, it was very hard to sit and wait for it to be over. When it was finally finished, I was able to relax. The surgeon informed us that the mass was not malignant, it was in fact a benign tumor called a meningioma. It was later confirmed by the pathology report.

We had crossed one bridge, but there were many more to cross. With a major surgery there were many possible deficits that could occur. Since the tumor was very close to the cerebellum, Eric had some impairments with his motor skills and balance. He was in the hospital longer than anyone expected. I watched him with pride when he worked with speech, occupational, and physical therapy. I even shaved my head after his surgery in solidarity when he was in rehab.

After 10 months, I was still worried about his progress because he was not back to his normal self. I wanted Eric to get a second opinion, but he believed everything would be alright. His walking was very inconsistent. Some days he would walk with the cane with no problems, other days he was hesitant to walk. I wasn't sure what was going on, I just prayed this would be temporary.

I've been in San Diego since 9/22/05, over a year. I wanted to play golf here, but figured I'll just wait for Eric to get better. I was worried he would fall if he was on his own. That's why I was here. I'm recently retired so I was able stay out here as long as necessary to take care of Eric. I went back home to Michigan every few months to take care of my rental properties and to go to my own doctors appointments. My wife usually relieved me of my duties for 1 week while I took care of my own business.

I know Eric will overcome all of his deficits in due time. I watch him working hard every day. He's really stubborn sometimes and tries to do things on his own. I go to the gym every day to work out with him. I lift weights and do cardio. He uses the bike and the treadmill, even though his PT doesn't want him to do it. All I can do right now is be supportive and make sure he doesn't do anything too crazy. Every father sees his own reflection in his sons. Oliver and Eric both turned out fine. I am very hopeful that things will turn out OK. With the help of God I will be able to come out from this experience a better person. My thanks go to all my friends and family for your prayers and support. God bless.

# I'll Be There

*Teresita Galvez*

I'll reach out my hand to you, I'll have faith in all you do
Just call my name and I'll be there
**-Jackson 5, *Ultimate Collection* 1995**

Whenever my son calls home, I am usually happy. He lives on the other side of the country. He calls on birthdays, holidays or if he needs something. September 10th, 2005, the day that Eric made "the" phone call, I suspected something was amiss. I heard his "hello and small talk," then silence. I thought we were disconnected. It took a long time for him to finally speak up. He told us about the MRI report and the large mass. He needed to consult with a neurosurgeon to have a craniotomy due to the size of the mass.

We were shocked. I did not really assimilate the graveness of the situation that instant. When it finally hit me, my blood pressure zoomed up. I was in a state of confusion, uncertainty, and disbelief. We wanted to go to him right away, but he thought he could handle all the pre-op procedures himself. He had many tests before the surgery: a CT scan, MRI, and angiogram.

Eric had a reaction after the angiogram. He was throwing up and was dizzy. His friend had to take him to the ER that evening. Joe decided to fly to San Diego the next day and stayed for the next 13 months with intermittent breaks whenever he needed to come home to take care of his business in Michigan.

In retrospect, I should have noticed a change in Eric's demeanor when he came home last August for a PT classmate's wedding. He lost some weight and looked haggard. He complained of a loss of appetite and occasional headaches. He lives a very active life. He's into surfing, marathons, and all kind of activities that young people participate in. He was like that ever since he was in school. He played many sports like baseball, basketball, track, wrestling, football, and tae kwon do. He and his brother both excelled in these sports.

My sister-in-law and I arrived in San Diego the day before the surgery. Eric was feeling a little better. He was given medication to alleviate some of his symptoms. The wait for the "day" was mixed with trepidation, insecurity, and fear of the outcome. I was glad his father was there to comfort and support him.

The day of the surgery was to be the longest traumatic day for all of us. It took a very long time. He was prepped at 5:00 am and we finally saw him in the ICU at 9:00 pm. I was not expecting it to be that long. It was a major surgery. A lot of things could go wrong. Being a medical technologist, I have seen instances arise during a procedure that could complicate things like, cardiac arrest, renal and respiratory failure.

I was already panicking. We were getting conflicting information from the volunteers and nurses. I know the surgeon and his associate were occupied, but there should have been at least one person who could come out from the OR to inform the relatives that the surgery was still in progress. You cannot imagine all the things that were going through our heads.

The hours passed. We were the only three people left in the waiting room. All this time I knew that my husband and his sister were having the same fears by just looking at them. Early in the evening, two attendants came and carried a body bag from the same wing as the OR site. Maybe that was where the morgue was. I was petrified, but then if something terrible had happened, we would have been told. That reasoning helped me from having a heart attack.

I stationed myself by the OR entrance asking anybody that came out if Eric was still inside. Finally the OR head nurse came out and told us that the operation was still in progress and would be finished in an hour or so.

We were only able to relax when he was transferred to the ICU. The surgeon was very optimistic. His initial diagnosis was the mass was a meningioma, a benign tumor. This was later confirmed by the laboratory report.

Eric could barely remember his stay in the intensive care unit. Since I was there from the very beginning I will try to fill the gaps. He looked awful that night after the surgery. His head was wrapped in bandage with tubes on both sides of his head and wires everywhere connected to all kind of monitors. He was heavily sedated. He recognized where he was when he woke up the next day. The staff asked him questions which he was able to respond correctly.

The third day, he wanted to get up and test himself to see if everything was okay. He is a very active person and not used to being bedridden. He was very restless and wanted me to take him home. He is very strong so the staff felt he might try to get up on his own; they had to restrain him, which made him more agitated.

When he was able to get out of bed and sit on a chair, they started to send the therapists to start working with him. The first question he asked was the outcome of the Michigan football game the day before. Saturday was football day; he watched it with a friend. He was having a good time cheering every time his team scored. He was out of bed sitting in the nearby chair. After a while he wanted to go back to bed. He was helped by the staff back to bed. While sitting on the edge of the bed, he fell backward. I just stood there motionless, not able to do anything. I wonder sometimes if the fall did any damage; the next day he complained of double vision and headache.

By Monday, he was getting hungry. He wanted to eat solid foods. The first request was pizza. The ICU nurse accommodated him and ordered one. We had to cut it into bite size to avoid choking. He was moved to the third floor of the main hospital for a night while the rehabilitation center was getting his room ready.

When he finally made it to the rehab center, the team of speech, occupational and physical therapists started him on a rigid schedule. He had problems with speech, balance, swallowing, and a lot of other deficiencies after brain surgery. However, his surgeon was very optimistic.

I wanted to believe him wholeheartedly. I am thankful the operation went well. We were now faced with a long road to recovery.

The ICU nurses, doctors, rehab social workers, his co-workers and everybody who took care of him were very helpful and supportive. Friends and relatives prayed for him and sent him moral support in the form of cookies and junk food. The people that know him well knew that he would enjoy sweet treats more than flowers. It has been almost a year since he was diagnosed with the brain tumor. Throughout this whole ordeal, Eric was always motivated and has held a positive attitude. He has persistently worked hard every day to get back into shape.

I came to stay with him a few times. I have noticed the gradual improvements he has accomplished: from the wheelchair, to the walker, now slowly walking with a cane. I hope and pray that he will be back to his old self. I know in my heart that he will be able to overcome these deficits and bounce right back with the help of God.

I am very grateful to everyone: family, extended family, friends, co-workers, even complete strangers who gave us their support and prayers. Above all to our Lord and all the saints I asked favors from in our hour of need.

# Friends' Perspectives

# Ain't No Mountain High Enough

*Mason Tassiviri*

Listen, baby
Ain't no mountain high
Ain't no valley low
Ain't no river wide enough, baby
If you need me, call me
No matter where you are
No matter how far

**-Marvin Gaye**, *Gold* 2004

H is name is Eric. But, he's also known as Deuce[1] and later, after hitting the big 3-0, we upgraded to calling him "Trey" to pay respect to his wisdom and years. But, for the most part, all his friends call him Galvez. Maybe it's a carry-over from high school – from the days of calling your teammates by their last names – or maybe it's because that calling him Eric doesn't quite do him justice. You might know a couple of different guys named Eric, but you have only one friend named Galvez.

Ask anyone that knows him, and you would hear the same descriptions: intelligent, optimistic, motivated, and caring. Ask anyone that just met him, and they would similarly describe him as athletic, good-natured, and shy. And, no…he sure doesn't look 30; you would have undoubtedly carded him if you were selling him alcohol. But let me try to describe him as I see him, a friend who is too humble to describe his positive traits himself.

It is very important for you to understand who he is and what he is like if you have any hope of understanding what he is experiencing, how this tumor has impacted his life, what his friends and family are

---

1   Nicknamed after his run in with the law…

observing and feeling, and for you to fully appreciate the context of his present circumstances. If you can picture yourself in his shoes, or be able to watch him as if you were present by his side or cheer him on or possibly even treat him, then you serve to benefit from this book. I hope it is successful in this endeavor as this will help you professionally, personally, or even better both.

There are certain people you meet in life that you really identify with, and Galvez happens to be one of those people for me. I relate to him on many different levels, many of which we have never openly discussed or discovered together, but which we share. That's part of the package. Galvez is not known to be a big talker unless you're watching ESPN together. For him to want to share his experiences with others is a perfect example of his nature. On the one hand, he's not an expressive, verbal, be-in-the-spotlight type of guy. On the contrary, he's so laid back and understated you might forget he's hanging out with the gang. Yet, choosing to use his experience and his recovery time to motivate, teach, and share with others is very much his style.

Galvez may be someone you might know…a son, a brother, a husband, or a friend…but he's not just some guy as he humbly presents himself…he's that rare breed of individual that rises above everything and gives you that rare glimpse of what people can potentially be: good. Not adequate, good. But, good in the sense that you would first think of him as an example of the best our humanity had to offer.

That's a lot of pressure, I know. If you ask me, it's an outright burden to be conscientious in this sort of way. But, you would never know if Galvez felt this burden. First, you would never be able to track him down. You could check the local gyms, the surfing spots, or his favorite running courses, and if you could keep up, you might find a small amount of time [in between gasps of air] to discuss it. His character and health make the tragedy of this tumor all the more devastating. Everyone wonders, "Why would this happen to Galvez of all people?"

I first remember hearing the whispers. Something was definitely up, but I couldn't put my finger on it. Some interesting gossip maybe?

I sensed something was happening before I understood what it was or who it was happening to. We were all gathered together, hanging out, when he pulled me aside. His demeanor was calm and cool but with something serious on his mind. He broke the bad news to me gently, considerate not to hurt my feelings. That's just like Galvez to care about how you might take the news. "Oh shit, oh shit, oh shit," I remember thinking to myself. Deep down, I was really hoping he was pulling my leg. But, with all the other symptoms he was reporting like the dizziness and the numbness in his face, I knew he was serious.

Galvez went on to tell me the operation would be scheduled sometime in late October and that he would appreciate keeping things on the down low until he could let everyone know in his own time. I remember feeling very guilty when I found out I was one of the last friends in our group to find out. Why wasn't I more available for him? After all, he spent the entire summer patiently coaching and encouraging many of us to run a half-marathon. I felt instantly panicked. If Galvez would have shown any fear or concern, or would not have been so composed, I would have surely lost it. My mom also lived through a brain tumor near her brain stem and I was flooded with all the memories and emotions of her experience that echoed in my childhood. I remember going home that night and confiding in my wife what I had learned. I cried uncontrollably that night for both of them, for the injustice and for the suffering of two people I cared about.

The surgery approached very quickly. It came much quicker than anyone could have foreseen in retrospect. It seemed like time fast forwarded up to the day of the surgery, and then seemed to hang forever in slow motion when waiting to receive the news. "How did it go? Is he okay?" We were all starving and anxious for information. We finally received confirmation from our friend Chris, the family spokesperson, that Galvez was going to be fine. We were all so relieved to hear the surgery went well. I felt compelled to visit him as soon as possible to show my support.

I visited Galvez after his surgery. I vividly remember the first time I saw him because the image will stay in my mind for a long time. I hope I will never have to see one of my friends in such a vulnerable state. I entered his room and found him sleeping in his wheelchair. He was slumped in his chair in the middle of the room next to his bed. My eyes immediately gravitated to his scar. I thank my friend, Lilly, for preparing me beforehand. The sight of the scar would have been hard to handle without the advance warning.[2] It was much larger and much more real than what you could have predicted. The scar was so fresh and raw that it was visually and emotionally cutting. It was at that moment that I realized that I didn't even have the slightest understanding of the magnitude or gravity of my friend's situation. Reality hit me very hard.

After standing in the room for what seemed like an eternity contemplating what to do, I decided to gently nudge Galvez to let him know I was there. He acknowledged me and we exchanged greetings. I felt embarrassed for waking him, but I wanted him to know that his friends were concerned about him. We spoke only briefly because he was obviously overpowered from exhaustion and medication. After I left, I decided I would visit him as often as possible.

I visited Galvez regularly in between his busy schedule of intense physical, occupational, and speech therapy sessions. He was constantly being interrupted and awakened in the hospital, and I remember him being so tired. I tried to make frequent but brief visits, so he wouldn't feel obligated to receive me. At the very least, I could speak and exchange pleasantries with his parents, who were faithfully by his side. I am sure that Galvez would have preferred to be left alone, if it wasn't for this temporary distraction I provided him by enjoying some time with his parents. I think he appreciated those brief moments of relief almost as much as he enjoyed the white chocolate macadamia nut cookies people would bring him. That's the other thing. Between the Krispy Kreme donuts, the cookies, and the other goodies people would bring him, we couldn't believe that all the junk food and decreased activity didn't cause a noticeable fluctuation in his weight. His metabolism and fitness

2    I can only imagine how Lilly must have reacted.

have always been extraordinary. I was certain that his conditioning and healthy lifestyle were going to be key to his successful recovery.

During my second or third visit, I started experiencing a lot of anxiety before entering the hospital. My throat would swell and my heart would race in anticipation. It is difficult enough to watch someone you care about go through this experience once, but I was instantly reminded of my mom's experience. Although I remembered the events surrounding her recovery, I was too young to comprehend the emotions of the experience. That was definitely not the case this time; I was overwhelmed.

After my second anxiety attack, I started asking my wife to come with me or tried to organize group visits with other friends. After all, what good would my company be if I'm more shook up than the actual patient? It almost makes me laugh when I think back on it. It also makes me only admire and respect Galvez even more for his courage. I never saw or heard him feel sorry for himself or show any discouragement, let alone fear. He remained focused on his therapy and diligent in setting goals to speed up his recovery. I would like to think that I was upset and anxious for both of us, but I couldn't take any credit for his resolve under stressful conditions.

At the beginning, Galvez showed tremendous progress. Every time we would visit him, he would get a little better. His motor skills improved tremendously in just a short time. He went from being completely bedridden to being able to stabilize himself to sit up and turn. He started to show improvement in his ability to use his arms and grasp things. His double vision and drooling diminished over time, eliminating the need to use his eye patch and increasing his confidence to speak. (These were important developments to help him regain a sense of normalcy.) But, I think everyone felt relieved when he started to get on his feet again. First, he began to stand up with some assistance and he quickly progressed to standing up using his own strength. We were so impressed when he began walking slowly[3] with the walker. He was doing absolutely great.

---

3    I can't emphasize the word *slowly* enough.

In fact, Galvez was doing so great so quickly, a lot of us expected to see him up and running after a few months. But, re-learning how to walk and regain his motor skills has developed more gradually than expected. A year later, Galvez has conquered the walker and has moved on to using a walking cane. Although his progress has been remarkable, Galvez continues to challenge himself. The next goal is to complete a 5K walk near the one year anniversary of his surgery. He invites his friends to join him on beautiful Sunday afternoons near San Diego Harbor to train with him. Regardless of whether people attend or not, you will find him there preparing. You will catch him checking his watch to see how long he has been walking or hear him set the landmark target to walk to in front of him. "I'm aiming for the third trash can" or "we're going to walk past the hotel and back." I really enjoy meeting up with him on these days because I am inspired by his goal setting. I wish I could take his skills and apply them to making me more productive in my own life. I guess I'll just have to wait for the motivational seminars to teach me the "how to" if I can't pick it up from observing him.

I feel fortunate to recount these thoughts knowing that my buddy, Galvez, will be able to read and appreciate them. The magnitude and impact of the surgery and the subsequent recovery were not well understood; I believe only now, a year later, people have begun to realize what a serious, life changing event this has been. Galvez is still determined to do everything within his power to rebuild his life from this interruption. He continues to set goals, motivate himself and train. He is by far his toughest critic, most ambitious trainer, and most valuable asset. His drive, work ethic and optimism are his greatest tools. I hope that patience and recognition of his progress and diligence will only increase his peace of mind and fuel his determination. I am proud of my friend for his character and will continue to encourage Galvez to be Galvez. What's the next milestone, brother? If you need me, just call me…

# True Colors

*Lilly Ghahremani*

But I see your true colors
shining through
I see your true colors
and that's why I love you
so don't be afraid to let them show
your true colors
true colors are beautiful
like a rainbow

**-Cyndi Lauper, *She's So Unusual* 1983**

Summers always go by so quickly, don't they? Usually they do, but not last summer, oh no. I got a little come-uppance for luring my friends to do a charity run with me 7 am one morning that spring. I crossed the finish line in a complete state of runner's high, and Eric leaned over and said, "If you like this, you should try the America's Finest City Half Marathon this summer with us." "For sure, sign me up!" I said, only half paying attention.

The next week when he started scheduling our training runs I realized what I'd gotten myself into. I'd give you the play-by-play of our summer of training, but I've already suffered, so why should you? Eric worked us so hard, using his fitness to motivate us time and again. Up hills, doing sprints, and running in the stifling heat of San Diego's hottest season.

A few weeks into training, Eric started asking me to check for traffic. Um, I was doing that already! But that's not what he meant. He wanted me to look both ways for him, because he would get dizzy if he did. So I did, and I enjoyed that he ran my pace because of his dizziness – it meant that we could talk about how hard it was in the dating scene and give each other advice on the dating battlefield. Once in awhile I'd ask him how he was feeling, but there's a fine line between being a caring friend and being irritating, so I soon stopped. Always positive, always encouraging, he trotted by my side for those few months.[1]

Before we knew it, the day of the race was upon us. This time Eric wasn't doing anyone any favors- he was going to run ahead of us and make good time. When I got to the finish line, he was already there, wearing his medal. He mumbled something about collapsing, but we were so high on success that he didn't make a big deal about it. Apparently he'd collapsed at mile 12 and the paramedics were on him. "Get off me! I want to finish!" he'd said. And he did. That's Eric for you.[2]

Life went back to normal, but then Eric mentioned to me that he was going to see a doctor. He started to confess different symptoms that he'd been ailing. Never a complainer, he had waited until he got worried. We went to the doctor together. Before walking in, he gave me a clipboard and a list of questions I was supposed to take notes about. Through the discussion with the doctor about the diagnosis and the details, I tried to write. Afterward, he critiqued my note-taking skills. I stood there in disbelief – all of this going on and he was under control enough to critique my handwriting? Were the notes even relevant? There was a tumor. He would need surgery. Things were changing.

I offered for my father to read his MRI again. Maybe there would be something that this doctor had missed. Like a little kid, you hope your parents can do something. They couldn't do anything, so they just joined the army of supporters Eric was building up.

The surgery came and went. I've never seen a friend in the hospital, and I hope to never see it again. Drugged beyond belief, the Eric we visited was a shell of his former self. It's always worse before it gets better, I reminded myself. The weeks flew by (for us, arguably not for him!)

---

1   And I was a good crossing guard, as evidenced by the fact that you're reading this book!

2   He *still* finished an hour before me. Sheesh.

We'd visit him and be silly – in those ways, things hadn't changed. He showed good humor when the nurses hovered around him deciding who they should set up with him. I was more impressed by Eric in how he handled himself than ever before. Being in a hospital is no fun, but visiting him was. We'd talk and joke and sit around and he always made you glad you came. Every time I saw him there was progress made. Maybe he looked like he'd put on a little bit of weight or he was speaking more clearly.

It was a bizarre world. Eric, the model of physical health, was suffering and there was nothing we could do to help him. That was the hardest part. Someone who is so willing to do things for himself wasn't able to just right now. However, with each visit, I was quickly set straight. There was a lot he could do for himself and he was damn well going to do it. I became more and more proud of him. I saw sides of him that I hadn't gotten to know that well before. It's so true that when someone goes through tragedy, their character shines through. In this light Eric was persistent, driven, sometimes stubborn ⊠ and always optimistic. "Can I help you?" "No, I can do it" echoed through our conversations more and more. He was able to accept help walking or getting something, but only when it was truly needed. Nowhere in the months of bedrest did laziness creep into his soul.

People don't have to be at their "best" for you to learn from them. Perfect Specimen Eric was just one variation of the person we have come to know and love. Every time I see him he looks better. It's such a relief to have him back home.

Circumstances will come into our lives that we cannot control. What we can control is how we react to them, no matter how devastating they may be. Everyone looks good in happy times. It's when things get tough that we see each other's true colors and really find out who we are and what we're made of.

# Jesus Walks

*Christopher Lum*

(Jesus Walks)
God show me the way because the Devil trying to break me down
(Jesus Walks with me)
The only thing that that I pray is that my feet don't fail me now
(Jesus Walks)
And I don't think there is nothing I can do now to right my wrongs
(Jesus Walks with me)
I want to talk to God but I'm afraid because we ain't spoke in so long

**-Kanye West**, *The College Dropout* 2004

My name is Christopher Lum but you can call me Chris. I was born and raised in Ann Arbor, Michigan. I just moved out to California a year ago and now I'm currently living in San Diego. I'm working as a consultant as a site developer. In other words, I play on the internet and create websites. It's seriously a fun gig (there are times of stress of course) but I love playing on the computer. Why not get paid doing the things that you love to do? I'm a big Detroit sports fan. BIG Detroit sports fan. You name it: Detroit Pistons, Detroit Lions, Detroit Tigers, Detroit Red Wings. Growing up in Ann Arbor, I learned to love the University of Michigan (GO BLUE!!) sports programs, especially football and basketball.

I've known Eric for as long as I can remember. We've been friends since around the 2nd grade. It's hard to remember when exactly we met or when we became friends but I've always felt a kinship with him because we are the same age and our younger brothers are the same age, as well (two years apart). I felt his pain when his brother would cause trouble because I went through the same thing with my younger brother. Although we went to different schools growing up, that didn't mean that we didn't see each other. Especially during the summer, we would hang out at Eric's parents house for family gatherings. Once we started getting older and heading into high school, we didn't hang out as much, which was expected since he was busy with school/football/wrestling/track and I was busy with school/marching band/symphony band/track. After high school, Eric went to Michigan while I went to Purdue and it was hard to see if our paths would cross again. God led me back to Michigan and there I would meet Eric again. After that, we became better friends. We've been through a lot together since then… parties, grilling, FASA (the Filipino American Student Association at U of M), serenading girls, friends getting married, the same friends having kids, moving, and now rooming together.

Finding out about Eric's diagnosis was shocking. When he was feeling sick, not eating, not working out as much because of dizziness, I thought that it was an inner ear infection like Eric had thought. I was surprised that he had to go get an MRI and even more surprised to find out he had a brain tumor! The word "tumor" is a very scary word, especially if someone you know says "I have a TUMOR." The worrying set in once I found out about the tumor.

It was definitely hard dealing with the fact that Eric had to get this thing out of his head. Seeing him in the SICU (surgical intensive care unit) was harder to take than I thought it would be. I spent so many hours praying to God and hoping that Eric was going to be fine. I remember the first time visiting Eric and seeing him with tubes in his head. It was scary to see. When you see a loved one like that, you feel helpless and you wish that there was some way to ease the pain. I cried walking out of the hospital. Eric is an athlete and when you see him like that, it's just hard. I would pray every day and go to mass in the mornings before work. I had to put my trust in God that He would help Eric fully recover. I had to be a point of contact while Eric was starting to recover and I felt like the answers I gave to people were not good enough. I felt people's need to want to help Eric and to be there for him. I felt everyone's helplessness. I was there in person to take on this burden of helplessness. Once Eric got into rehabbing, more people were able to visit him and for me, that made me happy and I'm sure it made Eric happy as well.

Eric has gone through a lot of therapy; I am not too worried anymore. It's still not easy seeing him not do the things that he would like to do. I'm sure that he would love to go out more, go surfing, and do all the things that he loves to do. I can tell that he wants to do things on his own without my help or his parent's help or anyone else's help. I want to help him but at the same time, I think that he wants to do it on his own. He's a physical therapist, he should know what he's doing. Eric's a fighter and he'll be fine. I trust in God that he will be fine.

# Believe

*Christopher Thompson, DPT*

If you want it you got it
You just got to believe
Believe in yourself
Cause it's all just a game
We just want to be loved

**-Lenny Kravitz**, *Are You Gonna Go My Way* 1993

"Want a chip?" This would often be my question to Eric when studying at night. We would be studying or working on projects, and like most college students, I would take a break for a snack. Often this would be a familiar brand of cheese-coated tortilla chip (I'm not in the business of selling a particular brand; I'm a physical therapist) and Eric would always reply, "No thanks, man." Wow, what willpower this man has! That was Eric, always taking great care of what he put in his body! Now, imagine how I reacted to the news of what was residing in his head besides that big ol' brain we're all so proud of. How could a person who takes such good care of himself have a tumor growth in his head? I lived with this guy and saw how he lived, there's no way he has a brain tumor! Not possible, no way! Then I thought, yup, anything is possible, we've read and studied about this sort of thing. Most of us have friends who have stories of "other" people who have had tumors and treatment, but now it was time to live it first hand. Well, I tried to share my cheese-coated tortilla chips and that didn't work, so I guess I will just have to settle for sharing my thoughts.

This first thing I remember was visiting with Eric in the Summer of 2005 in San Diego while on a road trip in California with some undergraduate buddies. Eric was talking of having episodes of dizziness and we discussed the idea of his new hobby of surfing and the possibility of water in his ear and a possible ear infection. Now, in physical therapy school we learned about balance, proprioception, and equilibrium in regards to the inner ear and your first thought goes to that, not a brain tumor! I suggested what Eric already knew, go to the doctor to get screened for an ear infection. At the end of our trip, we all met in Las Vegas for Eric's 30th birthday, and he informed me that things were actually getting worse than before. Ear infection, huh? After a while of being home and Eric going through a series of check-ups, he called me with the news. Then I thought, "Why couldn't it have been as simple as that ear infection?" Now, it's a whole new ballgame that we have only read about in textbooks and heard in lectures. The next event did not surprise me at all. Eric stood up, dusted himself off and asked, "What do we do to beat this thing?" In school we were taught to encourage our patients into being active and educated participants in their healing process. Now, Eric stood up and practiced what he preaches to his therapy patients. Eric always has been and always will be an active participant in his healing process. And I thought all of the learning experiences with Eric were over after graduation.

Now I look at life as a huge learning opportunity and everyone you meet has a role to play in that learning process. Eric has had his fair share of contributing to my education. Whether it was putting golf balls in the apartment while quizzing each other over material or reading over papers and projects with suggestions for improvement, Eric was always there to help educate me. I don't tell many this, but he also educated me on defensive basketball! Ask anyone who has had that gnat guarding them! You know what I'm talking about, you think you've lost him, then BAM, there he is again! He is tenacious that Galvez is! I don't think that tumor had any knowledge of this before setting up shop in his head. Galvez is tenacious and committed to his goal of recovery and that is a lesson that he shares with us all. I have always recognized a certain level of commitment from Eric to his family, friends, education, a healthy life and a job well done. It is when a person faces adversity and continues to have that same level of commitment, or even greater, that you truly take note and hopefully learn from his or her example. I thought that I had learned a valuable lesson after breaking my wrist last summer as far as being a patient, but Eric just had to go and out do me on that one! Well, Eric, I'm taking notes and I'm still learning. I'm just worried about how that might affect my student loan debt?

Now this whole experience has not only made me think about my relationship with Eric, but also with the relationships that I share with my patients everyday. The word that comes to mind when thinking of Eric as a patient and his attitude toward recovery is "believe." Many healthcare professionals might feel that that word is only important for the patient and it is only the patient who has to take full ownership of the word. When I think of Eric in relation to the word "believe," I can truly observe the dual responsibility that he has to accept. Eric must not only "believe" as a patient, but also as a physical therapist. In the patient to physical therapist dynamic, the patient often enters this relationship with a position of uneasiness and uncertainty. It is the physical therapist to whom they look for that first glimpse of "belief." A patient's first perception of "belief" is that all is well and trusts that the path to health is one that we will be able to follow. The treatment of a patient starts with the therapist's initial "belief" in the patient's ability to return to health. How is a patient to believe in the recovery process if that same belief is not shared by the physical therapist in charge of his or her care?

Those associated with Eric know that he is already strong both mentally and physically (he's a little Pocket Hercules!) and that this is largely because he takes ownership of the word "believe." If this whole experience does nothing to make him even stronger, then at least WE can all be stronger for sharing the experience with him. Thanks, Eric, for the lesson of "belief" and the power that it brings.

# Higher

*Alvin Borlaza*

Let's make our escape
Come on, let's go there
Let's ask can we stay?
Up high I feel like I'm alive for the very first time
Up high I'm strong enough to take these dreams
And make them mine

**-Creed,** *Human Clay* 1999

My name is Alvin Borlaza, a typical 32-year-old guy trying to balance career and family, while remaining a kid at heart. I am an only child, born in the Philippines to hardworking, generous and loving parents. My family immigrated to the U.S. in 1975 when I was a toddler and we have lived in Michigan since then, settling into a close-knit community made up of wonderful family and friends. Currently, I am a web developer with an IT company outside of Detroit, MI. I am a huge sports fanatic and have cheered on Detroit teams for as long as I can remember, especially the Pistons and Wolverines. I have a beautiful fiancée and eagerly await building a family and future with her. She lives in the Washington, DC area and I will be relocating to the east coast to join her in a few months. Having grown-up in Ann Arbor and the metro Detroit area my entire life, it's hard to picture myself living anywhere else, but I am excited and welcome the change.

I have known Eric for a long time – over thirty years. Our parents became close friends shortly after we arrived in the U.S. There are countless photographs of Eric and I playing together that precede both our memories. The earliest snapshot I have seen shows us riding together on an amusement park 'kiddie' ride. Little did I know that would be the first of many memories we would share over the course of our lives. From playing hide & seek in the basement when we were kids, to experiencing our newfound freedom in college, we were always there for each other. In fact, it's impossible for me to picture any part of my life without Eric – past, present or future. He's like a brother to me…

In September 2005, Eric called me from San Diego. Since he had moved out west, we made it a habit to catch up or just talk sports over the phone. I had no reason to think this call would be any different. Admittedly, he sounded tense that night, but I never could have imagined what he was about to share with me. For those who know Eric, they understand that he is a straight-forward guy. He is always honest and direct when breaking bad news.

"I have a tumor in my brain."

The sound of those words knocked the wind out of me. I felt as if I was hit with a body blow from Rocky Balboa himself. My stomach hurt. I couldn't move.

"They say it's about the size of a golf ball. I'm pretty sure it's benign, but I'll have to have surgery," he said matter-of-factly.

I didn't know what to do or say. How could he be so calm? All I wanted to do was freak out and ask the obvious questions of how and why. But that's how Eric is. He won't let you worry about him.

I was scared and frankly, a little bit in denial. A huge part of me could not wrap my mind around it. How could the most physically and mentally strong person I had ever known be diagnosed with this? How could this happen to Eric?

As I learned more about the surgery and let the news sink in, I realized how serious this all was. With every piece of new information revealed to me, my anxiety grew. There were a lot of risks with the surgery, especially because of the tumor's location in his brain. He could lose his hearing. He could permanently lose some of his motor skills. He could die. I wanted to cry, but what stopped me was Eric. Whether he knew it or not, he kept me sane. I figured if Eric wasn't worried, then I shouldn't be either. As I'd done many times in the past, I followed his lead and adopted his positive outlook.

During the days leading up to the surgery, I sensed Eric was beginning to worry, although he would never admit to it. He left personal messages on the blogs and websites of friends and made it a priority to spend time with everyone he could. It seemed he was making preparations for the worst case scenario. I found myself having to play the strangely unfamiliar role of being the calm and confident one. I had to push my own fears and doubts aside in order to tell him it would be okay. The truth was, as much as I wanted to believe that he'd sail through all of this, it was completely out of my hands. A couple days before the big day, we talked casually about the surgery. He let me know what was involved and how long it was expected to take. I think talking about the surgery in a clinical tone helped him deal with his fear. I admit that I felt a little better, too. It figures that during the most difficult time in his life, Eric was still a support for me. But I still worried.

My friends and I kept telling each other that he'd be fine. "Eric's a fighter. He'll make it through this with no problem." That's what we all needed to hear. However, deep inside, I was terrified. Eric is my best friend. I can't imagine what it would be like to lose him. So many questions ran through my head. Did I let him know how much he means to me? Was I a good enough friend? Maybe I should have called him to talk more often. I probably should have visited him more. I also experienced some frustration. Why did he have to have the surgery out in California? The University of Michigan hospital has some of the best neurosurgeons in the world. If he had the surgery here, he'd be closer to loved ones. Closer to family. Close enough for me to be there for him. Spiritually, I questioned God: "Why did this have to happen to Eric?" "What if he doesn't make it?"

The day of the surgery was a long one. The hours could not have moved any slower. Eric told me it would take about eight hours, so I watched the clock intensely. I don't know if I have ever prayed harder than I did that day. After the eight hours passed, I had yet to hear anything. Eric's parents were in San Diego with him for the surgery and recovery. His brother, Oliver, was at home in Michigan. In wanting to do something to help the situation, I gave Oliver a call to see how he was doing. I figured Eric would want someone to make sure his brother was okay. Oliver had as much information as I had already heard, "Eric's still in surgery. The doctors don't have any updates yet." I guess no news was good news at that point.

I visited Eric in December 2005, just weeks after his surgery. He was still recovering in the hospital. I hate hospitals. I always feel uneasy in them, but I looked forward to seeing Eric again and giving him a hug. I needed to see him in person, partly to convince myself this was all real, and partly to make sure he was okay. I was anxious as I walked into his hospital room. I didn't know how to act. What should I say? I wondered if Eric would be able to read the emotions on my face. It had been a few months since I last saw him. Should I hide any concern? Is he going to look different? What if our relationship changes? Looking back, some of those thoughts sound pretty ridiculous, but this whole experience was new to all of us.

My friend, Chris, tried to prepare me ahead of time for what I was about to see. Eric is arguably the most physically fit person I know. Despite his small stature, barely standing 5'5," he's a star athlete and pound for pound, the strongest guy around. I remember being shocked seeing Eric lying in bed. Rounding his left ear, there was a cool scar, but it was much larger than I expected. He was squinting on one side of his face since he had lost some feeling in his cheek. I couldn't tell if he was smiling or even happy to see me. His speech was impaired and he slurred a lot. The coordination that made Eric the first selection in our pick-up football games wasn't there anymore. He looked much thinner. His muscle mass had dwindled, most definitely the byproduct of being bedridden for two months. The left side of his body was partially paralyzed. He could barely even clap his hands, much less walk. This was an incredibly hard sight for me to take in. But then, we started talking.

After a few minutes spent chatting, I could see that Eric's personality was still there. We warmed up with some small talk. I was thankful there was a TV to break the occasional awkward silence. I had never felt uncomfortable in a room with Eric before. Maybe I just wasn't able to handle seeing him that way yet. I grew more relaxed as time passed. It helped that Eric's Dad and Chris were in the room too. I watched how they acted "normal" around Eric and realized I could do the same. We ended up talking sports and caught up with each other's lives. I knew then that Eric was still the same person, despite outward appearances. "Pre-surgery Eric" would not want to be seen as disabled, so I wouldn't treat or think about him that way.

By the time I left the hospital that December afternoon, I managed to work through some of my fears. I was optimistic about Eric's recovery. Sure, he looked different, but he was still the same person inside. I was just glad to see him. After all, less than two months earlier, I was terrified I would never see him again. But, despite the happiness and relief I felt, there was a sadness that came over me. All through 2005, I had been planning a surprise party for my then-girlfriend. It was to take place two weeks after my San Diego visit. Not only would we be celebrating her 30th birthday, I would be proposing to her in a room full of our closest friends. Walking out of Eric's hospital room, the reality set in that he would not be by my side during this quintessential moment in my life. We wouldn't have snapshots together from this event. Thank God we have the opportunity to take more in the future.

I have witnessed Eric's progress from afar. I receive periodic updates from him, his family, and Chris. Every time I see or speak with him, I find myself looking for some measure of tangible improvement. I watch him struggle as he works to gain his strength and balance back. I am unsure of how to help him when I see him tremble as he walks with his cane. Should I offer to help? In the end, I figure he has already reached several milestones on his own. Since I have only seen Eric twice after

I visited in December, I realize my urge to help him is a result of my own insecurity with regards to his struggles. He is fine; I am learning to be.

Since he started rehab, Eric has worked through several goals. He started off with getting in and out of his wheelchair on his own. Then he moved on to using his walker to get around and now, he is using his cane. I bet marathons are not too far off in his future. Occasionally, he pushes himself too hard trying to reach the next milestone before he is physically ready, and he falls. But he gets right back up on his own and works even harder to achieve the next goal as soon as possible.

Watching someone with Eric's work ethic motivates me to do bigger things. It's incredibly inspirational to see someone who relentlessly stands up in the face of a challenge, even after getting knocked down. This fire of quiet determination has always burned inside him, and it continues to radiate, affecting those who come to know him. I believe that this natural ability to inspire others by example, along with the lessons gained from the experiences he's going through now, will make him an amazing therapist with the ability to strengthen and rehabilitate his patients' physical bodies and their human spirit. Work with him. Talk with him. Witness him as he reaches new levels… Then be inspired to go higher.

# Three Little Birds

*Rosalia Machi Arellano MSPT*

Don't worry about a thing,
cause every little thing gonna be all right!
Rise up this mornin,
Smiled with the risin sun,
Three little birds
Pitch by my doorstep
Singin sweet songs
Of melodies pure and true,
Sayin, (this is my message to you-ou-ou:)

**-Bob Marley & The Wailers**, *Three Little Birds*, 1977

So we're at an after-work happy hour and instead of relaxing and enjoying his beer, Eric, the new guy, is discussing all of his test-taking and study strategies for the licensing exam. He's telling everyone what he's already done and what his plan is leading up to test day. I thought, "Man, he really has everything planned out, right down to the minute - a little type A, huh? Can't we just enjoy the fact that we're not at work?" But he was just so cute about it. So determined and focused that you couldn't help but root for him and absorb some of his nervous excitement. As the night went on, he had the attention of the entire table, including myself. Everyone was asking more questions and giving him lots of encouragement. No doubt about it, Eric's fortitude was contagious.

I've been a physical therapist for seven years and worked in several different settings. I've been in skilled nursing facilities, outpatient orthopedics, subacute hospital care, outpatient and inpatient neuro rehabilitation, and most of all, acute care. I've always been the type of person who needs to explore all options before committing to something. But even so, I've been known to grow tired of routine and am always up for something new and challenging, as long as I've got an action plan in place. Planned spontaneity, is there such a thing? I don't know, probably not, but I always feel the need for a plan (and sometimes even several back-up plans, just in case), even if it's a last minute decision. This little bit of type A in me inevitably played its role in the relationship that Eric and I developed.

In 2005 we both trained for the *America's Finest City Half Marathon*. I thought Eric would easily finish much earlier than me, so I was surprised to find him standing at the finish line. "Woo-hoo. Eric, Eric!" I was yelling for him before I got close enough to notice the expression on his face. He looked a little disoriented and as if he was about to blow chunks. "Eric, what the hell? Are you okay?" He told me (what I would later hear all too often), "Oh yeah, don't worry about me. I'll be alright." But then Eric said that he got really dizzy during the race and fell down as a result, and he also felt uncoordinated. I was shocked and worried, but he assured me everything was fine. Afterward, I told my friend about Eric falling during the marathon and how odd I thought it was. Sometime later, I got the news of Eric's tumor. I couldn't believe it.

I made an effort to not visit Eric immediately after his surgery. I didn't think he would remember me even if I did visit him and I really wanted him to focus on his recovery. I planned on seeing him during his inpatient rehabilitation after he had a routine in place and could handle a little more distraction. I also felt I was in this sort of limbo area of friendship - more than a co-worker, but not quite a friend yet.

The first time I went to see Eric, he was in his wheelchair. His Dad, who is super sweet and always friendly, was sitting by Eric watching his *every* move. Eric was ready to get back into bed and he didn't want to call the nurse for assistance and then have to wait. I asked if he wanted or needed a hand. "Oh no," Eric responded, "I only need minimal assistance to transfer now." He tells me not to worry and his Dad can help him. I looked over at his Dad ("Pops" as I call him) and he looked like a deer in the headlights. "Man!" I thought, "Once a physical therapist, always a physical therapist, right?" It's impossible to switch it off even though sometimes I wish I could, but it just doesn't work that way. I *had* to put in my two cents about transfer training. I *had* to take the opportunity to give a transfer training lesson, right? Pops was definitely asking for the help. I asked Eric what transfer style he was using and if it was okay to help Pops, especially since he was asking. Eric just wanted to get back into bed, so he reluctantly agreed. I was happy and I really wanted them to be safe and do things the right way. So, that's basically how it all began. I started to become Eric's friendly (or pushy) little nag. I suddenly found myself in this strange role of friend/ co-worker/mother hen/queen of the nags.

When I walked out of Eric's room that first night, I immediately burst into tears, muttering only a single four-letter word as I tried to grasp what I just saw. How does Eric still have so much impairment? I see patients on the daily post craniotomy and they couldn't care less about what just happened to them. They just care about getting out of the hospital and smoking a cigarette. And they do! With their head bandages, hospital gowns, and no problems. So why couldn't Eric be like that? Why wasn't *he* walking around asking all the nurses when he could finally go home? He was still requiring moderate assistance for his transfers and was super ataxic. I had to have faith that things would work out the way that they were supposed to.

After a lot more progress, when Eric was home and in outpatient therapy, I received an email saying that he was raising money for the National Brain Tumor Foundation by participating in a short race. It had his typical "no big deal, come if you want to, but no worries" tone. Eric's goal was to walk the race without his cane. Of course, I had to ask him how he was preparing for the race, who was helping him, and what was the longest distance he'd walked so far. "Don't worry," he says, "I'll be alright. I'm on only minimal assistance now with the cane." I thought "Awesome!" and told him I'd be there.

Eric ended up raising a ridiculous amount of money and earned the award for top fundraiser. He really didn't care too much about it at the time. He was focused solely on completing the walk without the cane. Despite him forgetting about all of the distractions and uneven terrain, and as fun as it was playing his motivation games, it ended up creating a lot more work for the both of us. Eric would get distracted and his balance would be shot. I could feel him getting tired, but he just kept saying he was fine and wanted to keep going. Every time he tried to hold a conversation with someone and walk at the same time, it took nearly maximum assistance to recover his balance.

We finally made it to the finish line. I was so sore for a week after the race, but I was so impressed by Eric's determination and will. I was again in this spot where I just wanted to be his friend but couldn't switch off my PT mind. I really wished Eric told me about the race and everything sooner. I could have tried to help him build up his endurance. I'm all for pushing the envelope and challenging goals, but let's be smart about it! But as always, Eric's response was "Oh, don't worry about me. I'll be alright."

Several months later, Eric calls me up and says "I'm doing something crazy. I want to do the Carlsbad 5000. You can come if you want and walk with me." Alright (remember, I can't switch off my PT mind), I ask him who is helping him train, what assistive device he's using, if he's sure he doesn't want to try the walker, and maybe he should use his wheelchair since he's never walked that distance before. "Oh, don't worry about me," Eric says, "I'll be alright."

There were so many distractions during the Carlsbad. Eric was just being a nice guy, trying to wave or smile to everyone we were passing. "Don't do that," I thought, "Just focus!" Dan and I were both helping out Eric a significant amount and had to stop frequently to give him rests. But he just wanted to keep pushing through and finish. We completed the race after three *long* hours and Eric made the news that night. "Go Eric!"

After that, I told Eric that if he ever wanted to do anything crazy like that again, he'd better let me know ahead of time because we were definitely going to train! Again, mother hen nagging about being safe. I wanted him to push himself, I truly did, but why not do it in a safe way? I bet his Mom would agree with me!

The following year, it was 2008 and Carlsbad 5000 time again. I made sure we trained that year. Eric's trunk strength had improved by an amazing amount. His ataxia was still a huge problem, but I couldn't believe how strong he had gotten and how he overcame some of the ataxia through sheer brute strength. He really was at minimal assistance with the cane this time. To account for uneven terrain and all of the distractions, we made sure we had a second person to help during the race. We ended up shaving-off over an hour from the previous year's time! Eric was much more focused and it showed. He even listened to me when I told him he couldn't wave to people unless we were stopped. I have to give Eric a lot of respect for putting up with me as I continually barked orders at him during the length of the race.

Eric had a reason bigger than himself for completing the Carlsbad. He wanted to send a message of perseverance and awareness. I was so proud. It must have showed too, but not in the way I would have liked. During the race, a woman mistook Chris (a friend of Eric's who was helping us) and I for Eric's parents. She cheered "Yay, Mom!" "Oh great," I thought, "They think I'm Eric's Mom." I even had some makeup on! It was a pretty hilarious moment. In all seriousness, though, I don't think I've ever felt as much admiration for Eric as I did when we finished the Carlsbad that day because he was reaching for a cause far beyond himself. He was trying to reach out to as many people as he possibly could.

Eric made the news that night. I think that's when I was completely sure he was going to be okay. Without even trying or knowing he was doing it, Eric found his higher purpose. He doesn't see it that way, but that's what makes it so great. People are drawn to him. His personality is caring, inspiring and inviting. He has the most generous and genuine soul. I'm sorry for being such a nag but I just can't help caring about this guy…but Eric, I know, I know, don't worry, you'll be alright!

# Healthcare Professionals' Perspectives

# Long Road

*Daniel DeBeliso PT*

I have wished for so long...
How I wish for you today
Will I walk the long road?
We all walk the long road

**-Pearl Jam *Live: 25-5-00 Palau Sant Jordi -- Barcelona, Spain* 2000**

I am a physical therapist; I have been practicing for a little more than eleven years. I work at a fairly large hospital in San Diego, with a wide range of patient care areas. As a PT there, I have been able to work in acute care, intensive care, skilled nursing settings, acute rehabilitation, and outpatient settings. I am Eric's friend, coworker, and, currently, his physical therapist.

Eric and I met when he started his first job as a PT in San Diego around a year and a half ago. We have in common our roots in Michigan - I grew up in Detroit, maybe a 45-minute drive from Ann Arbor, where Eric grew up. I wised up sooner than Eric, and moved from Michigan to San Diego when I was 17. I started college at San Diego State University, and graduated from PT school at Long Beach State University.

I tell Eric I went to college with "California girls." He counters by saying he went to a real college with a real football team. Touché... Eric and I reminisce about playing high school football for rival schools back in Michigan's Catholic League. I am quick to remind Eric that my school kicked his alma mater's ass my senior year. Unfortunately, Eric was still young enough to play Pop Warner that year.

While Eric is Mr. Orthopedic/Sports PT guy, my experience is more in neurological rehab. As one would expect, we talk shop a lot during our PT treatments. Our shoptalk is usually mixed with our

BS-ing about our favorite underachieving U of M teams and Detroit professional sports teams. (Is a Rose Bowl win, more often than once every thirty years, too much to ask?)

My situation (knowing Eric, working with Eric, being Eric's friend, his physical therapist) is a strange one. As a PT, I have treated plenty of young athletes Eric's age; I have never treated one with a clinical picture like his, with such significant deficits to work through. And I certainly have never been as close to any of my patients as I am to him. This was not too easy. Eric's other friends and family can be 100% cheerleaders, always there for support and help. That is sometimes an enviable position. I am one of Eric's biggest fans. I get to high-five him when he succeeds in rehab, masters a new skill, or achieves goals. I also have been treating him for eight months. We have serious discussions about his progress, realistic goals, his readiness for return to work, options for participating in races, his activities at home, and particular ways his parents should help him at home (he loves that). In these cases, I have to act as a professional, not necessarily as a friend. I have to tell Eric the truth, not what he wants to hear. I hope he will always appreciate my honesty.

When I found out about Eric's diagnosis, lots of thoughts occurred to me, just like the rest of the people he knows. Sometimes these thoughts were from a professional standpoint, some were as a concerned friend. Also, I have a lot in common with Eric, and I am only four or five years older than he is; I often wondered how I would manage if I was in his shoes. For instance:

- **When Eric was diagnosed, he showed us his MRI. His tumor is that big? His head does not look big enough to have something in it that size...**
- **He looks okay. He doesn't look like he has a brain tumor.**
- **Wow, Eric has the ultimate game face. He is so calm, cool, and collected.**

- **He is so optimistic about the fact he is having brain surgery to remove a massive tumor. To hear Eric tell it, the surgery will be so simple, his surgeon is practically going to cut a hole in his head, tip his head sideways, and the tumor will just fall out of his head. Eric's optimism definitely helped his family and friends deal with his news.**

After Eric's surgery, I went to visit him in the ICU. It was the day after his surgery, he was still on a ventilator. His head had a big post-op dressing on it. He had so much swelling, his head was huge, like a medium-sized watermelon. Eric started therapies (PT, OT and Speech Pathology) in the ICU a few days later.

Eric is lucky he has been such a good athlete his whole life. Being in such good shape was a good starting point because he had major physical challenges right from the start. I had never seen a patient so ataxic. He had no trunk control, he had no perception of midline, so he would rapidly assume a side bent position with any upright position. Any attempt to move his trunk or limb would result in a wildly ballistic movement, especially with his left side. This obviously left him with difficulty trying to eat, brush his teeth, or walk. (While Eric is much improved since the onset of these issues, this incoordination is still the main focus of his treatment as an outpatient.)

Over the next few weeks, Eric's medical condition improved; he moved from the ICU to the main hospital surgical floors, and to the Acute Rehab unit. He made gradual progress in spite of his severe incoordination. Across the board, every PT that interacted with Eric was amazed that he could function at all, considering his persistent motor deficits. That athleticism and competitiveness of Eric's has served him well; if he had slow recovery of coordination, he would compensate by "muscling" his way by, learning to walk with a walker with almost all his weight through his arms placed on the walker. When he tried to take a step to walk, he subconsciously (and accurately) decided he could not trust his feet to land anywhere near where they should, so his upper body became his safety net, supporting himself on any solid support he could.

He has spent months in outpatient physical therapy, relearning how to move his body, activating and strengthening some muscle groups here, learning how to relax overactive muscle groups there, to put together more normal postures and movements. He exercises in the gym to train his muscles and movements from head to toe. He uses a mirror during lots of exercises, to observe his movements, so he can learn to reproduce desirable movements, and avoid undesirable ones. He has used our partial body-weight supported gait training apparatus, in which a harness (like a parachute harness) supports some of his weight as he practices walking with help on the ground or on a treadmill. He has progressed from relying on a wheelchair, to a walker, to a cane, and to no assistive device, with a little help. Eric still has limited motor control, but it is much more manageable; he is able to step where he wants to most of the time. (Previously we likened his foot placement to throwing darts; for a long time, he wasn't even hitting the dartboard, now his feet are usually landing near the bull's-eye.)

Eric's apartment complex has a gym in it, so his avenues for exercise at home have really expanded recently. He has been practicing walking on a treadmill there, and he is getting better with his weight on his feet, and much less on his arms.

It has been nine months since Eric's surgery. He has made good progress in his rehab since then, in spite of his ataxia, vision problems, and bouts of intermittent dizziness. As Eric's friend and therapist, I am proud of his perseverance, hard work, his achievements in his recovery, and continued good attitude. He still is not as independent as he would like to be, in his self-care, his mobility, and his readiness to work and play. Eric still has a lot of work to do.

Eric's situation is quite poignant for me. I have really reconsidered much of what I do as a therapist, as a result of my interactions with Eric. Treating someone so ambitious, so educated, so enthusiastic about his life and his disability, and someone who so much reminds me of me, has really made me think about what I am doing with my patients and to my patients. Here are some conclusions I have come to as a physical therapist, and advice I would give to prospective PT's:

- **Be your patient's friend, but during therapy, be his or her therapist first.**
- **Tell the truth, in regards to treatment, progress, and realistic goals. Telling your patients what they want to hear does no one any good if what you say is not accurate.**
- **Listen to your patients; you don't always have to run the show. You will find out a lot about what you should be doing as a therapist if you shut up and listen for a little while.**
- **You are a professional; you are your patients' therapist. You are not their parent. You can provide your best advice based on clinical information. Your adult patients make their own adult decisions. Your adult patient's decisions have adult consequences like everyone else's.**

# Learning to Live Again

*Stacey Nelson MS OTR/L*

I burned my hand, I cut my face
Heaven knows how long it's been
Since I've felt so out of place
I'm wonderin' if I'll fit in.

**-Garth Brooks**, *The Chase* 1992

I t's not often that you walk into a room to do an evaluation and your patient tells you that he has right-beating nystagmus and ataxia. Eric and I did not know each other well before his surgery, no more than to say "hi" once or twice. We work at the same hospital, but when Eric began working there, he was on the acute floors, and I was working outpatient and inpatient rehab. While I'm only a few years older, I live east of San Diego, I'm married with a baby, have way too many animals, and run another non-profit program in addition to working as an OT at the hospital. So, considering all that, I'm not a part of that young, going-out-at-night therapist group at work! Our not knowing each other was one of the main reasons I would be working with Eric, though, to hopefully make it a little more comfortable for him to receive therapy from his colleagues.

When Eric arrived on rehab, he was still having severe vertigo and nausea, along with diplopia (double vision). I had been following his progress on the acute floors, so I knew he'd had a rough time before coming down to rehab. He required an extensive amount of assistance even to come up to sitting and to maintain his sitting balance at the edge of the bed, and was unable to find or maintain a midline position. He had severe ataxia, with very poor control of his left arm and leg. He also needed an extensive amount of help for all of his self-care activities

– dressing, showering, brushing his teeth, going to the bathroom, etc. When Eric went home, he had made progress but all of these things were still significant issues. He was primarily using a wheelchair, and was still needing help with most of his self-care.

Eric began outpatient occupational, physical, and speech therapy in December. This was the time he also began radiation, and we were worried how he would be able to tolerate intense outpatient therapy sessions along with the radiation. This was a part that hit especially close to home for me, as my husband had received a very similar course of radiation 2 ½ years earlier for cancer in his neck, and I was really concerned about how Eric would do. He got through radiation really well, though, except for his fatigue, and he managed to push his way through in therapy without taking a break.

Outpatient therapy is a time when issues often arise that weren't present in the hospital. Patients are at home, where a change in level of independence, disability and access issues, and changes in relationships with family and friends really become apparent. In OT, we deal with a lot of personal issues that can sometimes be difficult to bring up with family or friends, like bathing and going to the bathroom, and they are issues that can either leave a patient depressed or hysterically laughing. Luckily Eric was able to keep his sense of humor about it. I'll never forget how hard we laughed the day we were discussing ways to keep a towel around his waist after getting out of the shower, and the dangers of "naked walker walking!"

Eric's outpatient treatment was a challenge. Physically, he is probably the most complicated person I have ever worked with. We worked extensively on trunk control and symmetry, weight bearing for tone normalization in his left arm, and improving gross and fine motor control of his left arm, and often incorporated a mirror for visual feedback. We also worked on improving independence in activities of daily living (ADLs). Eric has come a long way, but the progress was slow – much slower than Eric or any of us expected. No matter how hard things were, it was rare for Eric to let frustration show. I think it was solely his determination and physical strength at times that allowed him to "muscle through" a movement or activity that neurologically it looked like he shouldn't be able to do.

Working with another therapist as a patient has been both challenging and rewarding. It's fun to have someone who understands what is going on and is able to explain what he is feeling. Eric understands the medical terminology and the reasons for treatment, which makes explanations much easier. At the same time, it was almost like having a very sharp student – I'd better be able to explain the reason for everything I was doing! I also felt like it was really important to give Eric choices in every treatment. While I had set goals and treatment plans, I tried to focus most of each treatment on what he felt he most needed to work on that day.

One difficulty in working with a coworker is the need to bring up things that are hard to hear. Eric was initially planning on being back to work in March, and had his mind set on that. At that point, though, he was still requiring occasional help just to use the walker, and had poor control of his left arm and leg. His other therapists and I were confused and frustrated with his insistent focus on returning to work as a physical therapist so soon, when he was not yet even independent in his own self-care or mobility. I sat down with him one day and we talked about adjusting his goals – not abandoning his goal of going back to work but focusing more on the more realistic, and at this point more attainable, goal of becoming independent at home. I think it was one of the first times the issue had really been pressed, and it had us both in tears. Talking about this with any patient can be difficult, but telling a co-worker he was not able to return to work on the timeline he had planned was definitely not something I had had to do before.

Eric has had plenty of frustrating and difficult times throughout his months of treatment, but he's always remained focused on where he wants to be. His hard work, optimism, and determination have been humbling and rewarding to me as a therapist and make me proud of him as a friend. My biggest challenge during his journey has been remaining objective and realistic about his progress as his therapist, while being supportive and encouraging as a friend. He still has a long road ahead, but he's shown us time and again over the last nine months that he has the strength and perseverance to keep walking down that road towards his goals.

# Kickstart My Heart

*Antonio P. Pablo OTR/L*

Ooo, ahh, kickstart my heart
I hope it never stops
And to think, we did all of this...
To rock

**-Motley Crue,** *Dr. Feelgood*, 1989

"**I** wonder who that patient is. He looks like someone who works here," I thought to myself as I walked down the physical rehabilitation corridor. I finished out my day, went home and thought about this mystery person while I helped my children with their bath, homework, reading and Xbox. I couldn't get him off my mind. Then, at work the next day, I saw him again. He was wearing reading glasses like the day before. Later that same day, I talked to the therapist who was working with him. "Who was the patient you worked with this morning, the young person?" I asked, "He looks like someone who works here." "That's Eric," he replied, "Eric Galvez." I started piecing together the information in my mind. I thought he might be related to one of the physical therapists I knew at the hospital since there seemed to be such a huge resemblance. Then, it finally hit me. "That's Eric!" I wanted to make sure I wasn't mistaken so I went to the mystery patient's room to confirm my guess. "Eric, is that you?" I asked. "Yeah, it's me," he replied. My eyes grew huge with shock. "A lot has happened over the last few months. I had a craniotomy for a golf ball-sized tumor in my brain."

My name is Tony and I'm an occupational therapist. Eric and I worked together at the same hospital in San Diego before he was diagnosed with the brain tumor. In fact, we were both hired around the same time. I would see Eric at the mandatory new hire meetings with the manager and occasionally on the acute floors. We even evaluated patients together a few times, but we were just co-workers.

Eventually, I stopped seeing Eric on the acute floors. When I worked with other physical therapists, I would ask how some of their colleagues were doing, especially ones who used to work with patients in the main part of the hospital. The word was that some therapists wanted to expand their horizons, so they would put in requests to work in other areas of the hospital, such as outpatient, physical rehabilitation and home health. When I asked about Eric, I was told that he had moved to another part of our campus. "Good for him. More power to him!" I said to my colleague. That was the last update I received about Eric, until I saw him escorted in a wheelchair to his room.

As I worked with my patients in the clinic, I would routinely glance over at Eric as he worked with Stacey, his therapist. At the time, it was very difficult for him to sit upright on his own. In addition, it was a constant struggle for Eric to place his left arm in a position to stabilize himself. I would see him constantly working on different tasks as I worked with my own patients. My rotation in physical rehabilitation ended during Eric's stay and I didn't have the opportunity to see him anymore. Eventually, he was discharged from the hospital and returned home. "I should have asked him for his e-mail," I thought. "I hope he's going to be okay."

Two or three months went by and one of my colleagues told me that I would be taking over treatment sessions for one of her outpatients. "Sure, no problem," I said, "Who is it?" "It's Eric," she replied, "Do you remember him?" "I do," I told her, "Fill me in on what you've been working on." I had the opportunity to observe Eric during one treatment session before I took over. The Eric I saw was in stark contrast to the man I remembered from a few months ago. He was walking with a front wheel walker and a cane, as well. He sat upright at the edge of the mat by himself. I was astonished at the progress Eric had made since I last saw him. He seemed very comfortable and confident. "Man, Eric, you're doing pretty well, aren't you?" I asked. "I'm doing alright, but I want to do more," he replied.

As I became more acquainted with Eric, I found him to be the most unassuming, humble man that friends and family described him to be. As with all my patients, I directed my interrogatives towards their occupational history, i.e. typical day, in particular, what they love to do. Eric is a triathlete, a wrestler and a martial artist, yet his gentleness never revealed these facts. I incorporated wrestling into our treatment sessions because Eric was a champion wrestler. He knew what I was shooting for when I had him do constant repetitions of "sit-outs" and "reversals;" together we stressed good control. Yet the main reason we incorporated wrestling was because it was personally meaningful to Eric. We talked about "banana splits," "figure fours," and Eric's favorite move, the "reversal" (shoulder dislocating reversal). Mr. Galvez, Eric's Dad, was present for all the treatment sessions (his parents are very supportive and loyal). He said that I would make a good wrestling coach. "Ha!" I barely made the varsity team at 135 pounds. I am definitely not a coach. Yet Mr. Galvez made me feel special with his kind encouragement. Eric, throughout all the workouts, didn't complain. He went from movement to exercise, exercise to movement, without ever asking for a rest break. If I didn't tell him to rest, he would do the next activity without a word. "No wonder he was a state champion back in the day. Eric has heart," I mused.

As we continued to meet for outpatient therapy, Eric outlined additional goals. "I want to walk again, I want to run again, and I want to surf again." Walking and running goals I would leave to Dan, another therapist of Eric's. Surfing, on the other hand, brought a smile to my face because it's something I love to do. So, I told Eric there were some stipulations if I were to help him surf again. "Before you surf," I told him, "you have to show me that you can swim. Once you show me that you can swim, you have to show me that you can balance on a surfboard and paddle it around the pool. Once you show me that you can paddle the board, you have to show me that you can sit on the board without falling. Once you can sit on the board without falling, if you fall off, you have to show me that you can find the board, pull yourself back onto it, and sit on the board again." Eric and his Dad nodded in agreement. "I'll find out what our pool hours are so we can get started with the swimming and paddling."

Before we had a chance to get into the pool, Eric's outpatient therapy sessions ended. I wanted to continue working with Eric but didn't know how to proceed. Dan informed me that he and Eric were scheduled to work-out together after-hours once a week. I talked to my wife and she was supportive of me working with Eric after-hours and Eric was agreeable, too. The pool was open on late Friday afternoons so that would be our time. Our physical therapy colleagues occasionally conducted treatment sessions at the same time, but we had the pool to ourselves the majority of the time.

Swimming was difficult for Eric. Timing the breathing pattern for freestyle took concerted effort. In the beginning, Eric could barely swim across the midpoint of the width of the pool. Our inside joke was that he surely didn't want to drink pool water, so he better learn to time his breathing and get to the other side of the pool. Eric progressed to swimming the length of the pool. During one workout, after four or five individual laps, he appeared to struggle to reach the pool wall. Mr. Galvez and I were walking along beside him as spotters while he swam. He was one foot away from the wall. A single stroke was all he needed to grip the wall edge and pull himself up. As Mr. Galvez and I looked on, Eric swam, but without forward progress. Since he didn't make it to the wall, we lifted him up above the water surface and guided him to the wall. "Dude, cough it up," I told him, "I know you don't like drinking this water." He coughed and we laughed. Eric has so much heart, such willingness to finish, that he will swim to the other side of the pool, often on one breath. He knows that we'll keep working on his breathing for freestyle. Nonetheless, as Dan and Stacey had intimated earlier, Eric continues to muscle his way through his rehabilitation.

Preparation for surfing went the same way. Eric started paddling training on a boogie board. This would provide Eric a primer for the end goal of paddling his own surfboard once again. Balance and paddling training with a boogie board is a little easier compared to a short or long board because more than 50% of your body is in the water with your legs acting as "floats." It was difficult for Eric at first. He had a hard time staying in the center of the board and flutter kicking at the same time. He started with laps across the width of the pool and gradually progressed to the length of the pool. Next up was the short board. I brought in a six foot, six inch tri-fin that I retired long ago. Surfboards of this length are easier to balance on and paddle compared to a boogie board, but may be more difficult to manage if your main surfboard is eight feet or longer. Since Eric surfed on his performance long board, the tri-fin would offer a little more challenge to his prone paddle and sitting balance. Prone paddling on the tri-fin was easier to Eric. He paddled the length of the pool several times during each workout. Moving from prone to sitting and actual sitting on the short board proved more difficult. We continued to work on prone/sitting balance with the short and long boards when Eric left for his book tour.

Eventually, we decided to concentrate on balance with a long board. Eric and I surmised that prone balance and paddling would be much easier on the long board due to increased board flotation. We were right. Eric made that board glide in the pool. I still have to fix the ding he put in the nose of my long board when he made a turn into the metal ladder.

Sitting was still difficult for him, even on the long board. As compared to our initial workouts, Eric made big strides. We started incorporating 'pop-up' exercises. He would lay prone on the carpet at home or the soft mat in the clinic. After a few paddling motions, he would 'pop-up' to standing in his natural surfing stance while I spotted him. Eric progressed to where I no longer had to provide as much facilitation as before, yet still required much practice.

Surfing by the summer of 2007 was Eric's goal. I told him that it was attainable, but we had to keep working on the swimming, paddling, pop-ups, and sitting. "You're doing pretty well," I told him, "But remember that doing these things in the ocean will be completely different." Eric and his Dad agreed. The day finally came when our busy schedules allowed us to meet at the beach. I brought the board that Eric practiced on at our work-outs. Theresa, our physical therapist colleague and Eric's surf buddy, also came out to participate. We walked with Eric to the edge of the ocean. The wind lapped against the glass-like surface of the water. The sky was blue and the rays of the sun blazed through the disappearing overcast. "You ready, dude?" I asked him. "Yep," he said. "Alright, strap on the leash."

We walked Eric into the water. He lay prone on the long board with Theresa stationed on the nose and me on the tail. The surf was no more than thigh-high. Although the whitewater was small, Theresa and I decided to float him out to the impact zone. "Eric, we're going to turn you around," I told him, "Theresa will go back inside to spot you. I'll stay here with you and push you into a wave, okay?" "Alright," said Eric. We floated in the impact zone and then I saw it. The two-foot high peeler made its way towards us. Nobody was on it. "Alright Eric," I told him, "Start paddling." He started to stroke. The wave came and caught me perfectly with a slap to the back of head. I pushed Eric into the wave as it peeled past me. "Paddle, dude, paddle!" I yelled, as I saw Eric's feet and the tail of my board go over the falls. As the wave crashed, I looked for him through, on, under the whitewater. While I ran towards shore, I caught sight of Eric cruising along towards the beach while he tried to stand up. "He caught it. Cool!" Eric cruised and tried to stand, cruised more and tried to stand again, and then down he went. His splash sprayed everything that was around him.

Theresa arrived first. I ran as fast as anyone could in the water. We saw the board, but not Eric. Theresa and I were standing in mid-thigh deep water as it receded. Then we saw him in the water as he attempted to stand. Theresa and I helped him up. He began to cough and gag as the saltwater dripped from his head. "Dude, are you alright? You okay?" I asked. With water dripping down his face, Eric replied, "This is the most fun I've had in a long time. Let's go again!" This guy has heart.

# Part III:
# Random Stuff

# Taking Care Of Business

Taking care of business every day
Taking care of business every way
I've been taking care of business, it's all mine
Taking care of business and working overtime

**-Bachman-Turner Overdrive,** *Takin' Care Of Business* 2000

I had a hard time accepting the fact that I was going on disability and would be out of work for an extended amount of time. It wasn't like I got into an accident or had done something crazy that put me at risk for injury. I had surgery for something that **had** to be removed.

Money was what gave me the biggest headaches. I was constantly worrying about how I was going to pay for rent, food, and other miscellaneous stuff. Luckily, California is a state that has "State Disability" (Medi-Cal) coverage. From my understanding, most states have some sort of State Disability benefits. Basically, what this means is that every 14 days, you get about 2/3 of your regular salary. That is almost as much as a regular paycheck after taxes. At work, it is similar to the coverage women get for maternity leave. I figured I should be alright financially until it runs out. After all, I wasn't planning on being out longer than a year.

After 6 months, I was eligible for "Long-Term Disability" through work. (A nice perk working for a large employer.) From my understanding the big difference between Long-Term Disability and State Disability is that Long-Term Disability is taxable and State Disability is tax-free.

To qualify for California State Disability you have to have a physician's signature on a few forms. The social workers and the human resources staff at work were extremely helpful with all my questions. The State Disability coverage becomes active when you first "declare" yourself unfit to work. I started the ball rolling before my surgery.

It really helped that I was able to take care of much of the logistical information and forms before the surgery.

My boss was extremely supportive and helped to extend my leave of absence to nine months. This was a big deal because after my sick time and paid time off had run out, I was responsible for paying for my own health insurance. At that point I could pay my insurance through work $40/month for coverage or if I was "unemployed" $360/month for COBRA Interim insurance. As long as I was still an "employee," I would pay the regular $40/month.

Initially, at the end of 5 months all of my work benefits such as health insurance and work seniority would run out and then I would be terminated. My parents were very set on my return to Michigan to complete my rehabilitation. But, I had other plans. I had already set my mind on just getting better and staying in San Diego so I could live my own life. To me, going back home would mean failure, a world of nagging, and people getting on my nerves. I figured I would do better in San Diego because I was more familiar with the health and legal resources in San Diego and I could take advantage of walking outside. Luckily for me, my continued health insurance did not cover the services I needed if I were to leave San Diego. *Aww shucks!* It looked like I would have to stay in beautiful San Diego to finish my rehabilitation. It wasn't hard to convince my dad to stay in San Diego a little longer and help me. I preferred doing my rehab here for continuity of care, and I believed I could do better on my own here rather than starting over with a new set of therapists back in Michigan.

Nobody knew I would be out this long. I had my leave of absence from work extended from 3/8/06 to 6/8/06 and then to 9/8/06. I'm very fortunate to have a supervisor looking out for my best interests. She said that my job was waiting for me when I was ready to go back to work. Whew... Another concern resolved.

I am by no means an expert on the logistical and financial burdens associated with rehab. It is really important for you to be in contact with the social workers along with your human resources department at work to help you out. You need them. It also helps to plan for the worst so you stay one step ahead of any potential problems. I was always thinking that things would work out and I would get better soon. "Parental concern" probably kept me grounded. As much as I didn't like it, my parent's "pessimistic realism" and nagging helped to keep me on top of what needed to be done.

After twenty-four months on medical disability, determined by your physicians, you become eligible for Social Security Insurance Disability (SSID). You must register for this early! DON'T WAIT UNTIL TWENTY-FOUR MONTH MARK THEN APPLY. *This is important to get before Medicare.* From my understanding, you are eligible only to what you have paid into it. After that runs out, then you are on your own. I was fortunate to work for an employer that provided long-term disability insurance. While most of my classmates opted for the larger starting salaries, I decided I wanted to work at the place that would give me the best opportunity to grow both personally and professionally. I was very fortunate to find a job that offered excellent benefits in lieu of a high salary. My reasoning was the money will be there later. After all, money was not the reason I got into physical therapy. I'd rather gain the experience, the opportunities, and the best benefits first. I followed my heart and I'm glad I did. Without that long-term disability, I never would have been able to stay in San Diego and accomplish all that I have so far.

Applying for Medicare disability is a very complicated process. Medicare is a federal or government healthcare program. Unlike some countries where healthcare is available to all citizens, you have to qualify for it in the United States. It is closely linked to Social Security benefits (retirement at age 65 or the disability 24 months SSID waiting period). You need a physician's signature to qualify for Medicare. There are agencies out there like HICAP (Health Insurance, Counseling, and Advocacy Program – a free service available for Medicare advice) that can explain it better and apply the rules to your unique situation. Medicare requirements are constantly changing so it is best to talk to a professional. Medicare Disability is not easy to attain. I have heard horror stories from other brain tumor patients who were deferred Medicare Disability because their impairments were not easily observable: short-term memory, concentration, depression, confusion, etc. These individuals oftentimes have to apply multiple times to qualify for Medicare. The fact that my impairments were "visually noticeable" accelerated the approval of my SSID application. I consider myself "blessed" that I have no mental impairments and I am extremely prepared for all the physical challenges I am up against. However, this does not mean I am an expert on the financial issues associated with rehabilitation. Social workers have a lot of knowledge in these areas. They should be consulted before making any major health related decisions to develop a solid financial strategy for a patient's medical situation. It is best to prepare your options before you have a medical procedure. I recommend consulting with the appropriate people (social workers, case managers, human resources professionals, family members, and others) about how you will finance your care/follow-up care and manage your post-procedure finances. It will save a patient and his/her loved ones a lot of unexpected stress down the road.

# Learn Yourself

And we've all got to learn ourselves
before we can judge some one else.

**-Beautiful Girls**, *Learn Yourself* 2004

I learned these lessons so you don't have to. The following lists are a few lessons (big and small) I've picked up along the way on my road to recovery.

## Lessons For Patients

1. **Tell the doctor everything.** – The little "symptoms" might add up to something serious. You might be able catch something before it is too late.
2. **Do your homework.**[1] - Knowing about your potential condition is half the battle. (10 points if you recognize where that little tidbit came from)
3. **Write down a list of questions for your doctor before you go in.** - Great to do when researching
4. **Bring at least one other calm person with you to the doctor's office to take notes.** - In case you miss anything, you might need another level head on your side
5. **Don't bring anyone with you to the doctor's office who might get too emotional.** – Choose your family members wisely. The news will be hard enough for you to take. You don't want to have to worry about taking care of anyone else.

---

1   My mom used to say this when me and my bro were watching the Public Service Announcements at the end of *G.I. Joe* the cartoon series because "*Knowing is half the battle.*"

6. **Talk to as many people as you can about your condition.**
   – Obviously you want to talk to additional healthcare professionals, but common everyday people can offer great advice about things you haven't even thought of.

7. **Make friends with the nursing assistants.** – They are the ones that answer your call light.

8. **Have a rehab buddy.** – Talk to people in the waiting room. Having a friend in the same boat as you makes it easier to cope with things. They understand what you are going through. It makes "bitching" about things more fun!

9. **Don't be afraid to open up to your therapists... you see them more frequently than your doctor.** – You can tell them anything and they can help you attack any problems you run into or at least direct you to the right people.

10. **Discuss your weekly goals with your therapist.** – You can take control of your own destiny.

11. **Don't get stuck in a rut... keep yourself busy.** – You are not magically going to get better doing nothing. I treated my rehab as my new job.

12. **Set mini goals every day and every week.** – A great way to monitor your progress.

13. **Expect the worst so you're prepared.** – Keeps you on your toes.

14. **You have to passionately WANT to get better.** – Actions speak louder than words.

15. **Use dark sheets when you go home for the first time.** - Your bed sheets tend to get dirty pretty fast.

16. **A string on the bathroom doorknob is really handy when closing the bathroom door.**

17. **Peeing with the bathroom door open is annoying to other people.**

18. **Be prepared to fall.** - You're going to fall. Be prepared. Don't be afraid.

19. **Make sure you do something physical every day.**- Stay active.

20. **It's good to get out of the house for something other then rehab.**

21. **Laugh at yourself.** - Laughing really is the best medicine, but know when to turn it off.

22. **Most of your improvements will happen on your own time with the home exercise program**. - Therapy sessions should be used to learn new exercises or techniques and to measure the improvements.

23. **Make the most of your "time off."** - This is your opportunity to read that book you've wanted to read or start that hobby you been meaning to start but didn't have the time for.

24. **It's OK to ask for help. Just don't rely on it.** – Don't let people baby you. You can do a lot on your own.

25. **Set your goals high and modify them as you go along… Keep your eyes on the prize.**

26. **Alone time is precious.** * Get it whenever you can. The bathroom was my favorite place to get away.

27. **Don't feel sorry for yourself.** - You've made it this far. Focus your energy on something else LIKE GETTING BETTER!

28. **Keep a journal/ Start a blog.** – Helps you monitor your progress and it keeps everyone updated on your progress. Be careful, though; anyone can read your blog. I got tired of mine because everyone knew how I was doing, but I didn't know what was going on with everyone else.

29. **Join a message/discussion forum from a national organization.** – You don't have to post a message, although the "locals" are usually very friendly and helpful. The forums are a great way to meet people who are experiencing the same things or who have gone through the same adversity.

30. **Don't dwell on the past, remember that the future isn't written.** – Focus on what is going on now. You control your own destiny.

31. **I'm not invincible.** - I wasn't at risk or even in the common demographic for a brain tumor. People can get sick at anytime.

32. **Be realistic, you may not do exactly what you want but at least can do something similar to what you want.**

33. **You'll need help to get through this.** - Your friends, family and therapists are good places to start.

34. **Learn to adapt the things you can do to the things you want to do.**

35. **As time passes, people will visit you only at their convenience.**

36. **Try new things; you will surprise yourself.**

37. **Curiosity is a virtue and can lead to great things.**

38. **The only thing limiting you is yourself.**

39. **Hope cannot be lost. You give it away under dire circumstances. The trick is holding onto it under dire circumstances.**

40. **With proper preparation and a good game plan, it can be done.**

41. **Winners have 2 things: definite goals and the burning desire to achieve them.** (from a poster on my bedroom wall)

42. **If you set your mind to it, you can accomplish anything. At the worst, you guarantee your best effort, which can still get you pretty far.** - I learned this back in 1985 watching *Back to the Future* and modified it throughout the years. I try to apply this to everything.

## Lessons for Healthcare Students

1. **Every patient has a story. Listen.**

2. **Involve a patient's family.** – They sometimes feel helpless. Empower them.

3. **Every patient is somebody's son/daughter, brother/sister, father/mother, uncle/aunt, friend/ co-worker.** - Try to remember this when our dealing with assholes. Somebody out there loves him/her or once loved them.

4. **The bathroom is the most intimidating place when patients go home for the first time.** – For me it was the combination of being naked and on my own. I was most worried about falling in there.

5. **Going to therapy is the highlight of the day for some patients that are unable to get out much.** - Make them want to come to therapy so you'll both enjoy the sessions. It's more fun working with someone who is motivated.

6. **Learn something non-medical about your patient.** - It humanizes them. I was always bad with names, but I always remembered the gentleman who used to tell me about his dog. I don't remember all the details of our conversations but I remembered HIM.

7. **Make every patent feel like he or she is your most important patient.** – It is really easy for patients to feel invisible.

# Conclusions (January 2007)

People continue to tell me "You're an inspiration." I always laughed it off because the real inspirations to me are the patients who face challenges greater than mine everyday. My story is only one of thousands of "inspirational" stories. If you sit down and talk to a person that has a disability, I guarantee you will find an interesting tale.

My story in particular is interesting because I became someone I've always tried to help. Through this whole ordeal, I've learned to appreciate the little pleasures in life like taking a walk on a beautiful Sunday morning or sharing a good hearty laugh with a friend or family member. The biggest lesson I learned was that how you react to a difficult situation will dictate how people around you will react. Everyone will follow your lead. I'm a goofball and dork, so that made people around me more comfortable. I am the same guy I was before the surgery. Of course you need a few people to turn to for support, but everyone else will mirror your reactions. As a therapist I now understand how frustrating waiting and slow progress can be! Communication with the patient and his family is essential. You don't have to be best friends with your patients, but a good therapist should be someone a patient can trust and confide in.

When I first found out about my brain tumor, I really didn't know what to think. Honestly, the only moments when I was unsure of myself were when the people around me were scared. I have a very "reactive" personality. I can't believe everything that I've gone through thus far. Waiting for surgery seemed like an eternity, but the rehabilitation seemed to pass faster because I always had my sights set on accomplishing a specific goal. I'm not perfect and certain things got on my nerves (especially the "coddling" and preconceived notions about my perceived disability.) I felt more comfortable when people treated me like a regular person, not like someone with "special" needs. I really appreciated the truthful feedback from my therapists. Sometimes their feedback was not what I wanted to hear, but it helped me readjust my goals to be attainable. Positive feedback was important to hear, but too much of it was annoying. Each individual will deal with life's challenges differently, but the drive to improve one's self is universal. I believe it is somewhere in all of us. The goals of a good therapist should be: to discover a patient's way of dealing with challenges, tap into his desire to improve himself, and adjust their treatment accordingly with emphasis on patient education.

Family and friends play a key role in the rehab process. They should be involved whenever possible. Whether it is helping with the home exercise program, education on a patient's progress, or goal setting... they cannot be left on the outside looking in. They are the ones that will be interacting with the patient every day. It seemed like I was out of the loop with my friends and family for so long. I really didn't feel like going out. I just wanted to work on getting better, almost obsessively. I'm glad my friends and family were there to drag me out; otherwise I would have been a hermit! Their role was huge in keeping me sane!

Right now I'm eagerly awaiting my return to work. I do realize that it may be awhile before I return to work as a physical therapist. I honestly believe that other doors will open for me. My story is not yet finished. I still have my whole life ahead of me. I still have a lot of things I want to do. A disability is not the end of the world, but an opportunity to enjoy the world in a different/unique way. If there is one message I have for patients and therapists it is **"Just Fight It!"**

**Eric Anthony Galvez PT DPT CSCS**

# New Conclusions (revised 2 years later)

Much has happened since the book was initially published. I am still learning a lot about the new me. I've been on TV a few times, have done some traveling, and have met some amazing people! It has been an incredible journey! I hope you somehow connected to the book. This book was all about perspectives. While my perspective as young brain tumor patient with a medical background is unique, I think that the perspectives of the people around me were just as important. The people surrounding a person that has to deal with a devastating diagnosis are easily overlooked, but should not be neglected. My family and friends are the ones who helped me realize I can still accomplish what I want. Even I am surprised at what has unfolded. I think I'm just starting, too! I continue to surprise others and even myself with some of the new ideas I come up with. I look in the mirror every morning and I recognize the face staring back at me, but when I look at his eyes there is something there that wasn't there before. It's a look of sadness, anger, and hope. **Hope** for my own recovery. **Hope** that someday another parent doesn't have to lose a child to a brain tumor or cancer. **Hope** that conversely, another child doesn't lose a parent. **Hope** that we don't have to lose another loved one to these horrible diseases.

That tumor has taken away a lot from me. It took away a promising career as a physical therapist (which I was just starting to love). It took away all my hobbies. It took away my independence. It has made it even harder to find the perfect girl. I've watched with envy most of my friends get engaged, married, and have kids while I relearn to walk/dress/ eat again. This thing was a "blessing?" I don't think so. It was more of an "awakening." I am still learning patience. I have also learned that I am capable of doing things beyond my wildest dreams. I have always been a late bloomer, so I am not as concerned with starting my family as much as my parents are. I'm still the immature, witty clown I was three years ago, just a little more patient and wiser. That tumor took away so much, but *it couldn't take away everything.* Through this whole journey I've never felt sorry for myself or ever let go of my **Hope**. The medical community couldn't give me the answers or options I needed so I created them myself. I choose to share my hope with you. Just promise to share your **Hope** with someone.

**Hope** is something that cancer or a stupid brain tumor can't take away. You can only lose it or give up on it under dire circumstances. The trick is to hold on to it under those dire circumstances. I will never give up mine. I choose to share it. My story still isn't finished and the new me is growing stronger. I don't think I have another book in me, so I challenge you to share your **Hope**. You don't have to write a book, but do <u>something</u>. Make the world a better place! Everyone will appreciate it. PEACE.

**Eric Anthony Galvez PT DPT CSCS**

# Part IV:
# Appendix

## *Appendix A: Mobility Impairment Simulation*

T his is a paper I wrote in Physical Therapy school. We were asked to spend one day in a wheelchair to get the patient experience. It really opened my eyes to the struggles of individuals with a physical impairment. Little did I know, it would prepare me for some of the psycho-social issues I would face as a patient.

Introduction

Spinal cord injury is one of the most common injuries in "risk taking" males ranging in age from 15-35. The purpose of this project was to understand the physical and interpersonal difficulties that are common in people with spinal cord injuries. I began the project at noon on Sunday, January 13, at Genesee Valley Mall with my colleague Chris Thompson. To my surprise, there was a sidewalk sale going on that day. Propelling the wheelchair through a crowded and busy mall would be a strong representation of some of the problems a person with a disability would face. I spent the afternoon in a folding chair with adjustable leg rests. It was an older chair with no seat cushion and armrests that were not adjustable. The leg rests felt comfortable at the level I found them, but the seat was far too wide for me. The chair was not an ideal fit for me, but I was very curious to see how things would unfold with this project.

Section I – Psychological component

After getting the chairs, Chris and I set off in separate directions. The first thing I noticed was that as I was propelling the chair, people would not make eye contact with me. I could tell that people were staring at me from a distance, but as I got closer to them they would look away. I got the most blatant stares from little kids. Immediately after getting the chairs and looking at the map of the mall, a little two-year-old boy ran up to the chair and started pushing on my wheel. His mother ran up behind him and instantly apologized for bothering me. She was pretty embarrassed and quickly pulled her son away from us. Most of the young children were not shy about staring at me, but I would occasionally catch elderly people trying to "sneak a peek." I first realized this in front of American Eagle. I was sorting through a rack of clothes, when I turned around and saw an elderly man quickly turn his head away from me. At first I thought nothing of it, but when I turned around again I caught him staring and quickly looked in another direction. This happened numerous times throughout the day. The strangest responses I got from people were from teenagers and people my age. Most of the teenagers walking in groups would ignore me, it was almost as if I meant nothing to them. Of course, being teenagers, they were probably in their own little world, but they didn't respond they way I thought they would. I was expecting to see more "curiosity" out of them because we were a little closer in age. There were a few that I did actually make contact with, although they were store employees.

When I first got into the chair, I did not seek conversation with anyone because I still felt pretty uncomfortable and self-conscious in the chair. In general, the only people who greeted me when I entered their store were the "adults." I also found that if I initiated a conversation with someone, he or she felt more comfortable being around me. I think the most important lesson to take from this interaction was that if I projected myself as someone who was comfortable with my situation, then everyone else should also be comfortable with me.

Section II - Barriers

The first store I entered was the electronics store, Babbage's. Video game consoles for the X-box and Playstation II were located on both ends of the doorway, so the entrance was extremely congested. In order for me to enter the store, I had to ask people to get out of my way. It was pretty funny because these kids were so entranced by the video games in front of them that I had tap on them to get their attention. Little did I know that this would be a common practice throughout the day. Of course everyone complied, but once in the store I noticed three particular barriers. First of all, I noticed that there were many items located on the higher shelves. There was no way I could reach them from my chair. Secondly, the aisles were very narrow so it was very difficult for me to maneuver my chair around the store. In addition, the store was very crowded because of the sidewalk sale, so that only made my maneuverability around the store even more difficult. Interestingly, none of the salespersons offered me assistance inside the store. It may have been because they were busy, but I was curious to see how it would be in the other stores.

The next store I entered was a men's store that specialized in suits and dress clothes. This store was not as crowded, and the racks in the store were easily accessible, although there were a few suits and shirts on higher racks. Two salesmen were sitting behind the counter talking. As soon as I wheeled into the store, I was immediately greeted by both gentlemen and asked if I needed assistance with anything. I went directly towards a stack of shirts; they both continued their conversation. I approached the younger one, and asked him for some help finding some pants. The older gentleman had an odd/snobbish look on his face and walked away. I assumed that he was wondering why a person in a wheelchair needed a pair of dress pants. The younger man took me to a rack of dress pants and began showing me the different styles. I explained to him that I was a college student looking for pants for a wedding. I didn't mention anything about the chair. He seemed much more comfortable dealing with me than the older gentlemen. This may have been because I approached him, but once he got into his sales pitch he seemed very comfortable. The dress pants in there were way out of my price range, so I thanked him for his help and moved on.

Next I went to Marshall Fields. Again, this store was fairly crowded. In front of the entrance, there many racks that made it difficult to maneuver the chair. In addition, there were people in the aisles looking at clothes so it was very inconvenient to ask people to move out of the way. Once inside the store, I immediately noticed that many of the displays were set on tables that were high off the ground. I couldn't see the styles on the tables, only the colors of the sweaters. I wheeled up to one of the tables, pulled a sweater off and quickly threw it back on top of the pile. I repeated this with 2 more sweaters until a salesperson asked if I needed help. He looked pretty annoyed, so I declined and then wheeled away.

I went into the GAP and tried to buy some boxer shorts. After some careful maneuvering, I found the right size and wheeled to the checkout counter. Upon getting to the front of the line, I had just realized how high the counters were. I took the wallet out of my pants for my credit card. I kind of laughed at myself because I could barely see over the top of the counter, and was signing the charge slip at chin level. Of course this was not that difficult of an activity, but I felt like a "little kid" looking up at everybody.

I continued the experience going throughout the mall, up and down inclines, through the smaller side stores, etc. The main barriers I found throughout the stores were layout (narrow aisles), high shelves and display tables, high checkout counters, and salespeople who were uncomfortable dealing with me. I had agreed to meet up with Chris in an hour, so I wheeled back to the center court and waited around. I knew he was going to be late, so I went directly into a sports memorabilia store and sure enough I found him there. We decided to continue our wheelchair experience and have lunch in the food court. Unfortunately, the food court was on the second floor so we had to take the elevator up. Getting on the elevator was not as difficult as I had thought. I worked as an aide at the U of M hospitals in Ann Arbor, so I was very comfortable being in the wheelchair. I had to pass a wheelchair competency test at work and was expected to be comfortable dealing with patients with spinal cord injury (SCI). My duties included basic wheelchair adjustments (adjusting leg rests, moving the tires forward or back, changing backs, etc.); teaching SCI patients how to perform wheelies/curbs; and teaching them how to propel their wheel chairs efficiently. Anyways, I went in the elevator first and waited for him upstairs. As I backed in, I noticed that although there was a line, nobody got on the elevator with me. I realized how isolated and alone some of our patients might feel. When Chris finally came up, I decided that I needed to wash my hands before we ate, so I wheeled over to the bathroom. I would go in first and wash my hands, Chris could then experience it himself. Unfortunately, there was no automatic door, so I had to push the door open and quickly push myself through the door. The sinks were very accessible, although there was not enough room for more than 2 wheelchairs. I did have a little difficulty pulling the door open, but quickly accelerated the chair through the door once I pulled it open. Coming out of the bathroom was not difficult because all I needed to do was pull the door open and pull myself through using the doorframe. I realized after all that work my hands were dirty again from touching the wheels and the door. Having clean hands was a lost cause. I waited for Chris to come out of the bathroom, and then we decided to eat and discuss some of the difficulties we had experienced throughout the day.

## Section III- Strategies

First and foremost, to address the issues of maneuverability of the wheelchair, I think that practice and comfort in the chair will only aid in the proficiency of maneuvering around obstacles. In addition, I think strategically picking days that are not as crowded may reduce the inconvenience of dealing with a crowded mall. I am not suggesting that people in wheelchairs should stay at home, but they perhaps should select times to go shopping when it's not as crowded, at least to start off. For example, shopping early in the day or later in the evening with an "assistant" would make this much easier. I think that once someone with a SCI is comfortable in his or her terrain, he or she should be able to do whatever he or she wants. For example, I've heard of SCI patients going "waterskiing" on lakes and playing wheelchair sports such as basketball or racing.

I was also surprised how uncomfortable those chairs really are, and how great the potential for decubitus ulcers. I remember performing pressure relief techniques at least once every five minutes. I have a very bony bottom, so I can only imagine the damage that could be done on the ischial tuberocities in people without sensation. That was the biggest surprise to me. I will be sure to preach to my future patients the amount of pressure I felt on my behind and the importance of pressure relief!!!

To address the issue of high tables or shelves, it would be very easy to recommend having an "aide" who might be able to bring things down, or even request assistance of a store clerk. In addition, the use of devices such as a mirror or some sort of grasping device could assist in looking at items high on shelves or in taking items off higher racks.

Finally, I think that when dealing with people who do not understand SCI, it is very important to make them feel comfortable with the situation. If you present yourself as comfortable with your situation, everyone will treat you accordingly.

## Appendix B: Ch-Check It Out

Check-ch-check-check-check-ch-check it out
What-wha-what-what-what's it all about
Work-wa-work-work-work-wa-work it out
Let's turn this, turn this party out

**-Beastie Boys**, *Solid Gold Hits* 2004

Once my vision improved after the surgery, I started reading more frequently. Some of the first books I read were accounts of patients with brain tumors. I read *Damn the Statistics, I Have A Life to Live!* by H. Charles Wolf and *Navigating Through a Strange Land* edited by Tricia Roloff. Both are great books. I found them online at Amazon.com. The first book was written by a successful guy from Ohio who had a glioblastoma multiform grade IV, the worst kind of malignant brain tumor. It details his first year with his diagnosis. The next book I read was a collection of essays written by different patients, family members, and healthcare professionals. I searched diligently for the accounts of young patients with meningiomas. I couldn't find any books.

The internet is a great source for general information, but not the definitive place for info. You should check your facts with your doctors. Websites like: www.emedicine.com and www.webmd.com are great resources for the common man for general information. For more detailed research, check out www.pubmed.com. I found the website for the National Brain Tumor Society, http://www.braintumor.org/. It was exactly what I was looking for. They posted their old newsletters online. In the newsletters, they spotlighted essays by patients with different types of brain tumors. I finally found the accounts of young patients similar to me that I was looking for! I am creating www.masskickers.com for the newly diagnosed and their loved ones. I have yet to find anything like it.

The following list is an excerpt from Tricia Roloff's book *Navigating Through a Strange Land*. It is a condensed and updated list of brain tumor organizations for patients to reference.

UNITED STATES – WEST COAST
The National Brain Tumor Society
West Coast Office
    22 Battery Street, Suite 612
    San Francisco, CA 94111-5520
    Phone: 415 834 9970
    Fax: 415 834 9980
Patient Services
    800 934 2873
Toll-free
    800 770 8287
E-mail: info@braintumor.org
Website: http://www.braintumor.org

Meningioma Mommas
9249 S. Broadway Blvd.
Unit 200-PMB#240
Highlands Ranch, CO 80129
Email: lindy@meningiomamommas.org
Website: www.meningiomamommas.org

UNITED STATES – EAST COAST
The National Brain Tumor Society
East Coast Office
124 Watertown Street, Suite 2D
Watertown, MA 02472
Phone: 617 924-9997
Fax: 617 924-9998
Email: info@braintumor.org
Website: http://www.braintumor.org

The Healing Exchange Brain Trust
186 Hampsire St, Cambridge, Massachusetts 02139-1320.
Tel: (617) 876-2002.
Website: www.braintrust.org
Email: info@braintrust.org

Brain Science Foundation
148 Linden Ste 303
Wellesley, MA 02842
Tel: 781-239-2903
E-mail: info@brainsciencefoundation.org
Website: http://www.brainsciencefoundation.org

UNITED STATES – SOUTH
The South Florida Brain Tumor Association
P.O. Box 770182, Coral Springs, Florida 33077-0182
Tel: (954) 755-4307

Miles for Hope
P.O. Box 5292
Clearwater, FL, 33758
Email: info@milesforhope.org
Website: http://www.milesforhope.org

Southeastern Brain Tumor Foundation
P.O. Box 422271, Atlanta, Georgia 30342
Tel: (404) 843-3700
Website: http://www.sbtf.org/

UNITED STATES - MIDWEST
American Brain Tumor Association,
2720 River Rd., Suite 147, Des Plains, Illinois 60018
Tel: (800) 886-2282
Fax: (847) 827-9918.
Website: http://hope.abta.org/site/PageServer
Email: info@abta.org

Fairview-University Brain Tumor Center
2450 Riverside Avenue, Minneapolis, Minnesota 55454
Tel: (800) 824-1953
Local Tel: (612) 672-7272
Website: www.braintumor.fairview.org

ENGLAND
The Brain Tumor Foundation
P.O. Box 162, New Malden, Surrey KT3 3YN, England
Tel: 0181 336-2020
Fax: 0181 336-2020

CANADA
Brain Tumor Foundation of Canada
650 Waterloo St., Suite 100, London, Ontario N6B 2R4
Tel: (519) 642-7755
Fax: (519) 642-7192
Website: www.btfc.org
Email: btfc@btfc.org

# Appendix C: Without Me

Now this looks like a job for me
so everybody just follow me
cuz we need a little controversy,
cuz it feels so empty without me

**-Eminem**, *The Eminem Show* 2002

This is my biography from my website www.ericgalvezdpt.com. I try to update my blog at least once a week. To find out what I'm up to now, check it out. There is some pretty interesting stuff on the website. Stop by and leave a comment.

I'm just a short Filipino-American guy from Michigan. I was a nerd in high school. "A's" filled my report cards and I still was into cartoons and science fiction. The only thing that kept me from getting picked on was the fact that I was good at sports. In high school, I was a first team, All-League defensive back in football, a state champion in wrestling, and a 4-year state qualifier in track. I was also an active member of the Student council and the National Honor Society.

In undergrad at the University of Michigan - Ann Arbor, I discovered beer, but somehow I was able to graduate with a Bachelor's of Science degree in Biology. Along the way, I helped to establish the first Asian-American interest fraternity in the midwest, was an officer in both the Filipino American Student Association and the Asian American Association, and joined an a capella group with no musical experience (it helped that one of my good friends was the director and that a lot of my friends were already in the group). After undergrad, I worked for 2 years as a physical therapy aide on the rehab unit at the University of Michigan Medical Center. I saw some pretty amazing stuff there. I really enjoyed helping people get better. After working there, I knew I was going to be a physical therapist.

I then moved to LA to go to school full time and improve my GPA before applying to grad schools. After a year in California, I moved back to Michigan to start physical therapy school at U of M-Flint. Before I left for LA, I applied to the U of M-Flint Physical Therapy Program since I still had my Michigan residency. I graduated from physical therapy school with a Doctor of Physical Therapy (DPT) degree in December 2003. I woke up one morning and decided I should move to San Diego. So I did. I've done the Michigan-California drive five times, three times with a companion and twice by myself. I knew 2 people in San Diego when I moved. I made some good friends in San Diego, but in the back of my mind I still missed everything and everyone I left behind in Michigan.

Things were going great in San Diego! I loved my job and all the outdoor activities San Diego had to offer. Then in the summer of 2005, I started getting intermittent episodes of dizziness, headaches, and nausea. I had an excuse for each symptom and would push through the symptoms to function everyday. I have always been the kind of guy who likes to push his physical limits. I learned how to swim just so I could go surfing and do triathlons. I completed two sprint triathlons and a half marathon in 2005. Like many other single men, I moved to the west coast from the midwest in the hopes of finding a sweet job, an active lifestyle, and a nice girl.

Nothing could have prepared me for the news I was about to receive. Brain cancer/tumors are pretty rare when compared to other types of cancer. On September 10 2005, I found out I had a huge brain tumor, a meningioma the size of a golf ball, on the tentorial membrane at the base of my brain between my brain stem and my cerebellum. The brainstem controls basic/unconscious body functions like heart rate, breathing, and facial/tongue movements. The cerebellum controls coordination and fine motor skills. Pretty important stuff at risk! I have a lot of friends here in San Diego, but I wanted to be with my family. The first people I called when I found out were my "Mommy" and "Papa!" I finally realized how much I loved my family. In the following months: I had brain surgery to have the tumor removed; radiation therapy to get rid of the remains; and Speech, occupational, and physical therapy for all the physical and mental impairments I was left with after the surgery. I was receiving rehab at the hospital where I used to work. In a strange twist, the people I used to work side by side with were now working with me as a patient!

As a patient I really wanted to be prepared for what lay ahead. My medical background helped immensely, but there were still a few things I wasn't ready for. I've been exposed to a number of patients with different diagnoses, but I couldn't find a book or other resource by a young single guy in the same boat as me. I was lying in my hospital bed and decided that when I got out of this, I would write a book… a "real" account of life as a patient for therapy students and younger patients with common situations and written in a style in which they could relate.

The rest of my story isn't written. All I know is that I'm going to fully enjoy living the rest of my story.

# Appendix D: Glossary of Terms

Many of the terms I describe in my own words. I would definitely double check any information with another healthcare professional. My definitions of certain terms are from my personal understanding and may not be completely correct. If you are writing a paper please cite another source for accuracy of the terms listed here!

**Angiogram** - An X-ray of blood vessels; the person receives an injection of dye to outline the vessels on the X-ray. (1)

**Astrocytoma** - A primary tumor that begins in the brain or spinal cord in small, star-shaped cells called astrocytes. (2)

**Ataxia** - An abnormal condition characterized by impaired ability to coordinate movement. (3)

**Auditory nerve** - Either of a pair of cranial nerves composed of fibers from the cochlear nerve and the vestibular nerve in the inner ear, conveying impulses of both the sense of hearing and the sense of balance. AKA vestibule-cochlear nerve, eighth cranial nerve. (3)

**Brain stem** – An important part of the brain that controls unconscious bodily functions like respiration rate, hearing, smell, heart rate.

**Cerebellum** – An important part of the brain that is responsible for balance and coordination.

**Chest X-ray** – An X-ray for the chest in my case to look for pneumonia or aspiration of liquids or solids into my lungs.

**COBRA insurance** - Continuation of benefits under a previous employer's plan after an employee leaves. Provides continuity of full care, but not necessarily affordable health insurance. Short term medical coverage is a COBRA alternative. (4)

**CSF (cerebrospinal fluid)** - Fluid surrounding the brain. It surrounds the spinal cord, as well. It acts as a cushion for the brain. It can be tested to diagnose neurological disorders.

**CT scan (Computed tomography)** - It takes cross-sectional pictures of different structures. Uses X-rays and takes about 5 minutes to complete.

**Doppler** - A diagnostic tool that uses low-intensity ultrasound to detect blood flow velocity in arteries or veins. (5) In my particular case, a Doppler was used to rule out a DVT.

**DVT (deep vein thrombosis)** – A blood clot in a vein, usually in the leg, which may cause swelling. If untreated, it can be a cause of death if a portion of the clot breaks away and reaches the heart. (6)

**Dynamic Standing Balance** – Balance when you are moving; i.e. walking or swinging a bat.

**ENT** – Ear, Nose, and Throat Physician.

**Extubation** – Removal of a breathing tube.

**Facial nerve** – Either of a pair of mixed sensory and motor cranial nerves that arise from the brainstem and divide immediately in the front of the ear into 6 branches innervating the scalp, forehead, eyelids, muscles of facial expression, cheeks, and jaw. (7)

**Foley Catheter** - A tube with an inflatable balloon at the tip used to extract urine from the urinary bladder. (8)

**Intension tremor** - A tremor during voluntary movements. It is the result of dysfunction of the cerebellum, in particular of the cerebellar hemispheres ("cerebro-cerebellum"), and is therefore part of the characteristic symptoms of cerebellar ataxia. (13)

**Mastoid bone** – A section of the temporal bone. (7)

**Meningioma** - A type of tumor that occurs in the meninges, the membranes that cover and protect the brain and spinal cord. Meningiomas usually grow slowly. (2)

**MRI (Magnetic Resonance Imaging)** - A diagnostic technique that provides cross-sectional images of the brain and other organs and structures within the body without X-ray or other forms of radiation. It takes cross sectional pictures of different structures. It is the most diagnostic tool for determining a diagnosis. (3, 10) The test takes about 60 minutes.

**Nystagmus** – Rapid movements the eyes when looking in a certain direction, sometimes indicative of a vestibular impairment.

**PICC line** – For blood draws and a way for administering medication. Usually placed in an arm. It is threaded from an artery all the way to the heart.

**PCP** – Primary Care Physician.

**Proprioception** – The ability to recognize the body's position in space.

**Semi-circular canals** – Any of 3 fluid-filled loops in the osseus labyrinth of the inner ear, associated with the sense of balance. (7)

**Swallow precautions** – There are different degrees of precautions. They are usually designated to post-surgical patients that have difficulty swallowing food or liquid.

**Temporal bone** – One of a large pair of bones of the lower cranium and containing various cavities and recesses associated with ear. (7)

**Tentorial membrane** – A membrane surrounding the brain.

**Tomotherapy** - A highly focused radiation therapy machine. It takes about 20-30 minutes to complete the whole procedure. Side effects for me were fatigue and patchy hair loss by week 4. (11)

**Tone** - The elastic tension of living muscles, arteries, etc., that facilitate response to stimuli. (11)

**Trigeminal nerve** – Either of a pair of cranial nerves essential for the act of chewing, general sensibility of the face, and muscular sensibility of the obliquus superior. The trigeminal nerves have sensory, motor, and intermediate roots and connect to areas in the brain. (7)

**Vasculature** – The blood supply to certain area of the body.

**Vent or ventilator** – A mechanical device used to facilitate breathing.

**Vestibular Nuclei** – The control center for the vestibulocochlear nerve, which controls hearing and balance. They are located in brainstem.

**Vestibular therapy** – A type of therapy that addresses dizziness by recalibrating loose particles in the inner ear.

**Wallerian degeneration** - It occurs at the distal stump of the site of injury and usually begins within 24 hours of a lesion. Prior to degeneration, distal axon stumps tend to remain electrically excitable. After injury, the axonal skeleton disintegrates and the axonal membrane breaks apart. The axonal degeneration is followed by degradation of the myelin sheath and infiltration by macrophages. The macrophages, accompanied by Schwann cells, serve to clear the debris from the degeneration. (12)

# References

1. www.spineuniverse.com/community/cancerdictionary.html

2. www.stjude.org/glossary

3. http://www.finr.com/glossary.html

4. http://www.assuranthealthshortterm.com/temporaryhealth insurance/short-term-medical/

5. http://www.brighamandwomens.org/vasculardiagnosticlab/terms.asp

6. http://www.spinal.co.uk/about/default.asp?step=4&pid=306#d

7. Anderson K, Anderson L, Glanze W. Mosby's Medical, Nursing, and Allied Health Dictionary, 5th edition. St. Louis: Mosby-Year Book, 1998.

8. http://glenlivet.mph.ed.ac.uk/endo/private/glossary.htm#sectionF

9. http://www.cis.rit.edu/htbooks/mri/inside.htm

10. http://www.sharp.com/hospital/index.cfm?id=2630

11. wordnet.princeton.edu/perl/webwn

12. http://en.wikipedia.org/wiki/Wallerian_degeneration

13. http://en.wikipedia.org/wiki/Intention_tremor